# Parenting
# Young Athletes

# Parenting Young Athletes

## Developing Champions in Sports and Life

FRANK L. SMOLL
AND
RONALD E. SMITH

ROWMAN & LITTLEFIELD PUBLISHERS, INC.
*Lanham • Boulder • New York • Toronto • Plymouth, UK*

Published by Rowman & Littlefield Publishers, Inc.
A wholly owned subsidiary of The Rowman & Littlefield Publishing Group, Inc.
4501 Forbes Boulevard, Suite 200, Lanham, Maryland 20706
www.rowman.com

10 Thornbury Road, Plymouth PL6 7PP, United Kingdom

British Library Cataloguing in Publication Information Available

**Library of Congress Cataloging-in-Publication Data**

Smoll, Frank L.
  Parenting young athletes : developing champions in sports and life / Frank L.
Smoll and Ronald E. Smith.
     p. cm.
  Includes bibliographical references and index.
  ISBN 978-1-4422-1820-8 (cloth : alk. paper) — ISBN 978-1-4422-1822-2
(electronic)
  1. Sports for children. 2. Parent and child. 3. Parenting. 4. Coaching (Athletics)
I. Smith, Ronald Edward, 1940– II. Title.
  GV709.2.S55 2012
  796.083—dc23
                                                                        2012017126

♾™ The paper used in this publication meets the minimum requirements of
American National Standard for Information Sciences—Permanence of Paper for
Printed Library Materials, ANSI/NISO Z39.48-1992.

Printed in the United States of America

# Contents

# 1

# You and Your Child in Sports

## Sanity and Madness in Competition

Dear Mom and Dad,

I'm writing this letter because you've always told me to tell you if anything was bothering me. This has been on my mind for a while, but I haven't been able to get myself to talk about it.

Remember the other night when my team was playing and you were sitting and watching? Well, I hope you won't get mad at me, but you kind of embarrassed me. Remember when I struck out with the bases loaded? I felt really bad about that, but even worse when I heard you yelling at the umpire. Actually, the pitch was a strike, but that pitcher is so fast I just couldn't swing. Then later in the game when the coach took me out in the fourth inning so Danny could play, I really feel bad that you got down on him because he's trying to do a good job. He really loves baseball and loves coaching us kids.

Dad, I know you want me to be a good ballplayer like you were, and I really do try as hard as I can. But I guess I just can't measure up to what you want me to be. The way you act when I don't do good, it makes me feel like I've let you down. On the way home the other night, neither of you spoke to me. I guess you were pretty sore at me for messing up. You made me feel like I never wanted to play baseball again.

Even though I'm not very good, I love to play and it's lots of fun being with the other kids. But it seems like the only time you're happy is when I do really good—even though you told me that playing sports was supposed to be for fun and to learn the game. I want to have fun, but you keep taking the fun away. I didn't know you were going to get so upset because I couldn't become a star.

This is really hard to say, and that's why I have to write it to you. I used to be really happy that you came to our games. Some of the kids' parents never show up. But maybe it would be better if you stopped coming so I wouldn't have to worry about disappointing you.

Love,
Chris

Chris's letter leaves little doubt that his parents are having a real impact on his youth sport experience. Unfortunately, it is not the kind of effect that one would wish for him. Perhaps Chris's parents are lucky, for their son has the courage to give them feedback on something that is bothering him deeply and influencing his enjoyment of sports. Maybe they can change their behavior, after realizing how they are unintentionally becoming a source of stress rather than a source of support. Like all parents, they want the best for their child, and they may honestly feel that they are supporting him in his sport activities. It also seems clear that there needs to be a change in their attitudes and behavior, if sports are to bring Chris and his parents closer together and his parents are to contribute to his enjoyment of the activity.

This book is for you, the parent of the young athlete. We wrote it because we believe that sport participation has great potential for improving the growth and personal development of children and for enriching the family. Because sports are so important to youngsters, what parents do and say in relation to athletics can have an important long-term impact. This book provides information that will help you make your child's sport experience constructive and enjoyable!

Parents can be a source of support, or they can create stress for young athletes.

All parents do as well as they can, within the limits of their awareness. We believe that the information in these pages will increase your awareness of, and help you deal more effectively with, the many problems and opportunities that can arise in youth sports. We welcome the opportunity to increase the knowledge of parents who have a strong background in sports as well as those who have relatively little athletic experience.

## THE GROWTH OF YOUTH SPORTS

How big are youth sports, and how did they get that way? Sports for children and adolescents in the United States actually go back to the early 1900s. The first programs were established in public schools when it was recognized that physical activity was an important part of education. Over time, sponsorship and control of some sports have shifted to a variety of local and national youth agencies. These programs have flourished, and today more children are playing than ever before.

> Youth sports are deeply rooted in our social and cultural heritage.

How fast have youth sports grown? Very fast! Little League Baseball, one of the oldest programs, is a good example. It originated in 1939 in Williamsport, Pennsylvania, as a three-team league for 8- to 12-year-old boys. The program was so popular that it spread rapidly. In its 50-year anniversary season, there were some 6,800 chartered leagues in 25 countries. Little League now encompasses a huge patchwork of nations and cultures, including Israel, Jordan, Russia, Germany, Japan, Canada, Australia, Poland, Mexico, China, Venezuela, and South Africa. As of the 2008 season, nearly 2.6 million 6- to 18-year-old boys and girls participated in Little League Baseball worldwide, including approximately 400,000 boys and girls registered in Little League Softball.

> An amazing number of youngsters participate in sports.

Programs in other sports have also shown rapid growth. Today more opportunities to play a greater variety of sports exist than ever before, particularly for girls and young women. Current estimates indicate that more than half (approximately 68 million) of the young people in the 6-to-18-year age range participate in agency-sponsored sports (e.g., Little League Baseball, American Youth Soccer Organization, Boys and Girls Clubs) and in school-sponsored athletics. This situation has required the involvement of increasing numbers of adults. Accordingly, millions of men and women volunteer their time as coaches, league administrators, and officials. And millions more serve as paid professionals in school-sponsored athletics. As programs have become more highly organized, parental involvement has also increased. Thus, in moving from sandlots and playgrounds to the more formalized organizations that now exist, the youth sport explosion has touched young people and adults in escalating numbers.

What factors have contributed to the rise of youth sports?

- Over the years there has been a clear recognition of the importance of wholesome leisure-time activities for children and adolescents.
- The expansion of large cities has decreased the amount and availability of play spaces.
- Many authorities have correctly looked to sport programs as a way of reducing juvenile delinquency.
- Sport has become an increasingly central part of many cultures and personal lives. People generally have become more fitness-minded, and the mass media have brought sporting events into the homes of countless numbers of families.
- The final factor accounting for the growth of youth sports is the most important one: Sports are an enjoyable and rewarding pastime. The most essential reason for participating in sports is that they can and should provide fun and enjoyment!

Growth in the popularity and scope of youth sports and in the role that they play in the lives of young people is undeniable. But this expansion has generated ongoing and, at times, bitter debate.

> Serious questions have been raised about the desirability of youth sports, and answers to the questions are not simple.

## SPORTS FOR CHILDREN AND ADOLESCENTS: THE DEBATE LINGERS ON

We have already identified some of the reasons for the rapid growth of youth sports. Obviously, this growth could not have occurred if adults did not believe that participation is beneficial. Those who favor such programs emphasize that there are many aspects of the experience that contribute to personal development. Some supporters have pointed out that sports are miniature life situations in which the participants learn to cope with many of the important realities of life. By playing sports, athletes learn to cooperate with others, to compete, to deal with success and failure, to learn self-control, and to take risks. Important attitudes are formed about achievement, authority, and persistence in the face of difficulty.

Adult leadership can be one of the truly positive features of youth sport programs. Knowledgeable coaches can help children acquire physical skills and begin to master a sport. Higher levels of physical fitness can be promoted by such guidance. The coach can become a significant adult in an athlete's life and can have a huge positive influence on personal and social development. Likewise, the involvement of parents can bring families closer together and heighten the value of the experience for young athletes.

> Sport programs for children and adolescents have both desirable and undesirable features.

On the other hand, youth sports have more than their share of critics. Coverage by the media is dominated by attacks on sport programs. Because mistreatment of children is newsworthy, sport abuses are likely to be sensationalized and widely publicized. Distortions frequently occur. One prominent sport psychologist spent 90 minutes with a reporter. For 80 minutes he discussed the positive aspects of sport programs, and for 10 minutes he talked about the problems in youth sports. The newspaper article dealt only with the problems. Furthermore, it misquoted the expert as saying that all sports should be eliminated for children under the age of 16. The media's overemphasis on the negative has understandably made some parents question the value of youth sports.

Undoubtedly problems can arise in sport programs, and some of these problems have been the focus of severe criticism. *Newsweek* once published a thoughtful editorial by former Major League Baseball pitcher Robin Roberts, titled "Strike Out Little League." The Hall of Famer pointed out that playing Little League Baseball can potentially place excessive physical and psychological strains on youngsters, and that programs sometimes exist more for the self-serving needs of adults than for the welfare of children. Experts in child development have claimed that adult-supervised and highly organized programs can rob children of the creative benefits of spontaneous play. They suggest that children would benefit far more if adults simply left them alone to their own games and activities.

---

**Even the very best programs have some faults.**

---

Many complaints focus on the role of adults in youth sport programs. Critics have charged that some coaches are absorbed in living out their own fantasies of building sport dynasties, and that consequently they show little personal concern for their athletes. Likewise, opponents of youth sports maintain that parents live through their children's accomplishments and place tremendous pressure on them to succeed. When coaches and parents become more focused on themselves than on the quality of the children's experience, something is certainly wrong!

The negative involvement of adults in sports has been linked to such problems as the inappropriate use of drugs for training and conditioning purposes, physical injury due to excessive training and competition, and blatant cheating and dishonesty. The *Los Angeles Times* reported that one misguided coach injected oranges with amphetamines, then fed them to his 10- to 12-year-old football players to get them "up" for a game. The *Washington Post* carried a story about a mother who forged a phony birth certificate for her 17-year-old son so that he could star in a league for 14-year-olds.

Who's right? Are youth sports a symptom of a serious, widespread social disease? Or are they the salvation of our youth? The answer is neither. No reasonable person can deny that important problems do exist in some programs. Some of the criticisms are well founded and can be constructive. On the other hand, surveys have shown that the vast majority of adults and children involved in sports find them to be an enjoyable and valued part of their lives. The bottom line is that sport programs are what we make of them. They can become a source of joy and fulfillment in the life of a child, or a source of stress and disappointment.

A realistic appraisal of youth sports includes recognition of their positive and negative features.

We believe that sports have a strong positive *potential* for achieving important objectives. The question is not whether youth sports should continue to exist. They are firmly established cultural institutions. If anything, they will continue to grow in spite of the criticisms that are sometimes leveled at them. The real question is how parents can help ensure that participation in sports will be a positive for their children.

What can you do to help achieve the many desirable outcomes that are possible? Perhaps the key to unlocking the potential of youth sports lies in being well informed about their physical and psychological dimensions. We hope that the information presented in this book will assist you in your role as a successful youth sport parent.

## THE RIGHTS OF YOUNG ATHLETES

When youngsters enter a sport program, they automatically assume responsibilities. But they also have rights. Adults need to respect these rights if young athletes are to have a safe and rewarding sport experience. In the United States, the National Association for Sport and Physical Education organized a Youth Sports Task Force and charged it with developing a "Bill of Rights for Young Athletes." The rights identified by these medical doctors, sport scientists, and youth sport administrators are presented in the box below.

We believe that the "Bill of Rights" provides a sound framework for fulfilling adult responsibilities toward young athletes. These rights will

---

### BILL OF RIGHTS FOR YOUNG ATHLETES

1. Right to participate in sports.
2. Right to participate at a level commensurate with each child's maturity and ability.
3. Right to have qualified adult leadership.
4. Right to play as a child and not as an adult.
5. Right to share in the leadership and decision-making of sport participation.
6. Right to participate in safe and healthy environments.
7. Right to proper preparation for participation in sports.
8. Right to an equal opportunity to strive for success.
9. Right to be treated with dignity.
10. Right to have fun in sports.

be dealt with in greater detail throughout the book as we explore their implications for enriching the sport experience.

## GOALS AND MODELS IN SPORTS

What do you want your child to get out of sports? What are the goals that you would like achieved? Parental objectives can range from simply providing a worthwhile leisure-time activity for children to laying the foundation for becoming an Olympic champion or a professional athlete. There are, of course, many other goals that may well be more appropriate. Some of them are physical, such as attaining sport skills and increasing physical fitness. Others are psychological, such as developing self-discipline, respect for authority, leadership skills, competitiveness, cooperativeness, sportsmanship, and self-confidence. These are many of the positive attributes that fall under the heading of "character."

---

The greatest contribution that sports can make to young athletes is to build character. The greatest teacher of character is on the athletic field.

—*Tom Landry, Pro Football Hall of Fame coach*

---

Youth sports are also an important social activity in which children make new friends and acquaintances and become part of an ever-expanding social network. Furthermore, sports can serve to bring families closer together.

Whatever your objectives may be, it is important that you become aware of them. And you must realize that none of these objectives can be achieved as a result of mere participation in sports. Simply placing a child into a sport situation does not guarantee a positive outcome. The nature and quality of the program, which are very much dependent on the input of adults, are prime factors in determining benefits.

Unlike youth sports, the major goals of professional sports are directly linked to their status in the entertainment industry. Former Dallas Cowboys wide receiver Peter Gent recalled that at the end of rookie

camp, a meeting was held to explain the responsibilities of a professional athlete. "The man to give the best advice was the team's public
relations director," Gent said. "He told us, 'Boys, this is show business.'"

In the *professional model* of sports, the goals are to entertain and,
ultimately, to make money. Financial success is of primary importance
and depends heavily on a product orientation, namely, winning. Is this
wrong? Certainly not! As a part of the entertainment industry, professional sports have tremendous value in societies around the globe.

> **Professional sports are a huge commercial enterprise
> where success is measured in wins and dollars.**

In the professional sports world, players are commodities to be
bought, sold, and traded. Their value is based on how much they
contribute to winning and profit-making. They are the instruments of
success in competitions and at the box office, and they are dealt with as
property or as cogs in a machine.

Professional athletes are often glorified by the media to create an image intended to generate interest and draw paying customers to competitions. However, many professional athletes feel that little real concern is
shown for them as human beings or contributing members of society. For
example, several professional teams have reportedly turned deaf ears to
reports of drug abuse by star athletes as long as the athletes continued to
perform well. In Lawrence Taylor's book titled *LT: Living on the Edge*, the
Pro Football Hall of Famer wrote the following about his battle with co-
caine addiction: "If they wanted to bust me, fine. But I knew they weren't
going to do that, not as long as I was who I was and my game was intact."

---

All they seem to care about is what you did for them yesterday and
what you can do for them tomorrow.

—*Willie Mays, Baseball Hall of Fame player*

---

The professional coach's job is to win. Those who don't usually
join the ranks of the unemployed rather quickly and unceremoni-

ously. No gold watches for years of service, either! A win-at-all-costs philosophy is required for advancement and, indeed, survival. Professional coaches do not receive bonuses for developing character. Their primary function is to help the franchise to compete successfully for the entertainment dollar.

Kids are not pros! The *developmental model* of sport has a far different focus. As its name suggests, the goal is to develop the individual. The most important product is not wins or dollars but rather the quality of the experience for the child. In this sense, sport participation is an educational process whereby children and adolescents can learn to cope with realities they will face in later life. Although winning is sought after, it is by no means the primary goal. Profit is measured not in terms of dollars and cents but rather in terms of the skills and personal characteristics that are acquired.

> In a developmental model, sports are an arena
> for learning, where success is measured in terms
> of personal growth and development.

Sometimes, the two athletic models get confused. We are convinced that most of the problems in youth sports occur when uninformed adults erroneously apply a professional model to what should be a recreational and educational experience for children. When excessive emphasis is placed on winning, it is easy to lose sight of the needs and interests of the young athletes. This common mistake is referred to as the "professionalization" of youth sports.

We asked earlier what you want your child to get out of sports. Perhaps we also should know about the objectives that young athletes seek to achieve. Scientific surveys conducted in the United States and Canada have indicated that young athletes most often list their sport goals in the following order of importance:

- To have fun.
- To improve their skills and learn new skills.

- To be with their friends or make new friends.
- For thrills and excitement.
- To win.
- To become physically fit.

---

**What does your child want out of sports?**

---

Concerned parents should ask their young athletes what *they* want from sports and why *they* wish to participate. Parents should not be guilty of forcing their own aspirations upon their children. Rather, you should make sure that young athletes have a say in determining their own destiny.

It is important to note that the primary goal of the professional athlete as well as many adults—winning—is far less important to children. In one of our own studies, we found that teams' won-lost records had nothing to do with how well young athletes liked their coaches or with their desire to play for the same coaches again. Interestingly, however, success of the team was related to how much the children thought their parents liked the coaches. The children also felt that the won-lost record influenced how much their coaches liked them. It appears that, even at very young ages, children begin to tune in to the adult emphasis on winning, even though they do not yet share it themselves. What children do share is a desire to have fun!

*Fun.* A term we use a lot. But what is it? Certainly, it's easy to tell when people are having fun. They show it in their expression of enthusiasm, happiness, and satisfaction. We've asked many children why sports are fun for them. Perhaps the most basic reason was given by an 8-year-old girl, who said, "Fun is when I'm doing something that makes me happy just to be doing it, like playing tennis." In other words, much of the fun in sports comes just from performing the activities themselves. One child played on a soccer team that almost never won matches. Yet the youngster could hardly wait for the coming season. Why? Because he had fun. He simply enjoyed playing soccer. Being with others, meeting challenges, feeling the drama of uncertain outcomes, becoming more skilled, all of these add to the fun of doing for doing's sake.

Certainly, winning also adds to the fun, but we sell sports short if we insist that winning is the most important ingredient. In fact, studies have shown that when children were asked where they'd rather be—warming the bench on a winning team or playing regularly on a losing team—about 90 percent of them chose playing over winning. The message is clear: The enjoyment of playing is more important to children than the satisfaction of winning.

The basic right of the child athlete to have fun in participating should not be neglected. One of the quickest ways to reduce fun is to begin treating kids as if they were professional athletes.

---

It's a disgrace what we're doing in the United States and Canada. We're asking kids to compete to win. Why not ask them to compete to have fun? We're trying to build our own egos on little children.

—*Sparky Anderson, Baseball Hall of Fame manager*

---

Perhaps most importantly, we need to keep in mind that young athletes are not miniature adults. They are children and they have the right to play as children. In fact, we all do. The Dutch historian Johan Huizinga wrote that to play as an adult, one must become a child again. Youth sports are first and foremost a play activity, and children deserve to enjoy sports in their own way.

Now, we are not suggesting taking away the uniforms or changing the team names. The youngsters enjoy these trappings. What we are emphasizing is the need to make sure that youth sports remain *child-centered* and do not become adult-dominated.

## PARENTS' ROLES AND RESPONSIBILITIES
Two important sets of adults combine with the child to form the *athletic triangle*. They are, of course, parents and coaches. The relationships that

exist among the points of the athletic triangle go a long way toward determining the quality of the sport experience.

Being a point in the athletic triangle implies both rights and responsibilities. When your child enters a sport program, you automatically take on some obligations. Some parents do not realize this at first and are surprised to find what is expected of them. Others never realize their responsibilities and therefore miss opportunities to help their children grow through sports, or actually do things that interfere with their children's development. In a sense, this entire book is about parents' roles and responsibilities. For now, however, we want to summarize some of the more obvious ones.

> The right of the child to participate in sports
> also includes the right *not* to participate.

Although parents might choose to encourage participation, children should not be pressured, intimidated, or bribed into playing. In one research study, athletes who felt "entrapped" reported less enjoyment and lower intrinsic motivation and benefits of being involved in sports and were more likely to drop out of sports. Even more profound and long-lasting are the effects that feeling forced can have on parent-child relationships. Just how profound is shown in the following statement made by a 40-year-old man: "If it hadn't been for sports, I wouldn't have grown up hating my father."

It is possible to be very supportive of a child's athletic interests without placing demands or pressures on the youngster. For example, National Hockey Hall of Famer Bobby Orr was fortunate in having very supportive parents. He recalls, "My parents bought my equipment, drove me to the rink, rubbed my feet when they were cold. I can't remember them saying that I was going to be a professional hockey player."

Parents should be observers and supporters of their athletically inclined children, but never pushers.

—Wayne Gretzky, National Hockey Hall of Fame player

Although coaches have the most direct contact with children within the sport environment, parents also involve themselves to varying degrees. Some parents assume an extremely active role, and sometimes their behavior and the demands they place upon children become a great source of stress for the child. Consider, for example, the following experience described by a youth coach:

> One night last season my team lost a close game. I sat the whole team on the bench and congratulated then for trying, for acting like gentlemen. I said I couldn't have been prouder of them if they had won. Most of all, I said, it is as important to be a good loser as a gracious winner. As I talked I could see their spirits lifting. I felt they had learned more than just how to play baseball that night. But as I mingled with the parents in the stands afterward, I was shocked to hear what they were saying to the boys. The invariable theme was, "Well, what happened to you tonight?" One father pulled out a notepad and went over his son's mistakes play by play. Another father dressed down his son for striking out twice. In 5 minutes the parents had undermined every principle I had set forth.

It is natural for parents to identify with their children to some extent, to take pleasure in their triumphs, and to suffer in their defeats and disappointments. The love bond that exists between parent and child virtually guarantees this process. Like all good things, however, this process of identification can become so excessive that the child becomes an extension of the parent. When this happens parents may begin to define their own success and self-worth in terms of how successful their child is, as in the following cases:

> Justin's father never was a good athlete. Now in his adult years, he is a "frustrated jock" who tries to experience through Justin the success he never knew as an athlete. Justin is pushed to excel, to put in long hours of practice, and to give up other activities. When he performs poorly, his father becomes withdrawn and gloomy. Dad takes home movies of Justin during practices and games, and visitors to the home are promptly shown some of Justin's triumphs. Justin himself is a reasonably good athlete at

age 12, but he is unlikely ever to become a superstar. In fact, a school teacher has become very concerned because Justin "doesn't seem himself" and is lagging in his schoolwork. The family's physician is concerned even more, because Justin has been complaining of abdominal pains and the doctor is fearful he may be developing an ulcer.

Nicole's mother was a champion collegiate swimmer who won a bronze medal in the Olympic Games. It is clear that the mother expects Nicole to follow in her footsteps. Nicole was a "water baby" at 6 months of age and was "in training" by age 4. She shows every sign of becoming a high-level competitor in her own right. She is now 10 years of age and has won countless medals in age-group swim competitions. Her mother clearly is delighted with and totally engrossed in her athletic development. But her father is becoming worried. Lately, Nicole doesn't seem to enjoy swimming as much. Last week she announced that she wanted to stop training and go to summer camp with some friends for several weeks. Her mother flatly refused to consider this, and Nicole burst into tears, saying that she didn't want to swim anymore. Nicole's father is concerned that her mother is placing so much pressure on the child to excel that she is experiencing burnout.

Justin and Nicole are showing clear signs of the stress caused when parents try to live through their children. Justin is being pushed to become the great athlete that his father always wanted to be, and Nicole is having to measure up to the standards set by her mother as a champion athlete. These children *must* succeed or their parents' self-image is threatened and the children themselves are threatened with disapproval or loss of love. Much more is at stake than a mere game or swim meet, and the child of such a parent carries a heavy burden.

> Parents can be a potent source of athletic stress when they overidentify with their child's performance outcomes.

At some level both Justin and Nicole must be aware that their parents' happiness depends upon how well they perform. Children are accustomed to being dependent on their parents and are often unequipped to handle a reversal of the dependency relationship. This is especially the case when the parent is demanding winning results rather than the best effort of which the child is capable.

We should point out that sports are not the only activities in which this may occur. The performance arena may be in academics, music, dance, or social popularity—any activity that has social or personal importance for the parent. But because of the importance of sports in our society, and particularly in the world of many parents, there is special potential for the dependency-reversal process to occur in the realm of sports.

One of the most important responsibilities of child-rearing is the role that parents play in shaping their children's perceptions and understanding of their world. Sports can be a proving ground for later life experiences. Therefore, you have the opportunity to help your young athlete accurately interpret and understand sport experiences and place them in a proper and healthy perspective. For example, you can play a key role in helping your child understand the significance of winning and losing, of success and failure. You can help your child define his or her success in terms of effort expended instead of the score at the end of the competition. Moreover, winning or losing a competition may be the result of external factors beyond the child's control, such as officials, weather, other players, or luck. Or it may be the result of internal causes, such as the child's ability and effort. By helping children to accurately interpret the causes of sport outcomes, parents help youngsters view the world more realistically.

There are other important challenges that must be met by youth sport parents. To contribute to the success of a program, you must be willing and able to commit yourself in many different ways. The following questions serve as important reminders of the scope of parent responsibilities. You should be able to honestly answer "yes" to each one.

### Can You Give Your Child Some Time?

You will need to decide how much time can be devoted to your child's sport activities. It may involve driving children to and from practice;

going to your child's games, meets, or matches; and assisting the coach. Many parents do not realize how much time can be consumed by such activities. Some parents who expect sport programs to occupy their child's time and give them more time for themselves are shocked to find that they are now spending more time with their children than before.

> Youth sports are *not* a free babysitting service!

Conflicts arise when parents are very busy, yet are also interested and want to encourage their children. Thus, one challenge is to deal honestly with the time-commitment issue:

- Ask about your child's sport experiences.
- Make every effort to watch at least some competitions (games, meets, matches) during the season.
- Never promise more time than you can actually deliver.

### Can You Accept Your Son or Daughter's Triumphs?

Every child athlete experiences "the thrill of victory and the agony of defeat" as part of the competition process. Accepting a child's triumphs sounds easy, but it is not always so. Fathers, in particular, may be competitive with their sons. This process is the opposite of the overidentification discussed earlier. For example, when Jack played well in a basketball game, his father pointed out minor mistakes, described how other players did even better, and then reminded his son of even more impressive sport achievements of his own. This reestablished his role as a dominant parent and thoroughly deflated Jack.

### Can You Accept Your Son or Daughter's Disappointments?

Disappointments are also part of sport, and they may be keenly experienced by your child at times. Would you be embarrassed if your child broke into tears after a tough loss or after making a mistake? Could you put your arm around and comfort your child at such a moment?

Can you tolerate becoming a target for your child's displaced anger and frustration when there is no other outlet for disappointment and hurt? When an apparent disappointment occurs, parents should be able to help their children see the positive side of the situation. By doing this, you can change your child's disappointment into self-acceptance. Again, emphasizing effort rather than outcome can be an important means to this goal.

### Can You Show Your Child Self-Control?

Conduct at practices and during competition can have an important impact on your child. Parents who yell at or criticize athletes, coaches, or officials set an incredibly poor example for their youngsters. You are a significant role model for your child in all aspects of life, including sports. It is not surprising to find that parents who exhibit poor self-control in their own lives often have children who are prone to emotional outbursts and poor self-discipline. If we are to expect sportsmanship and self-control from our children, we need to exhibit the same qualities in our own behavior.

---

There is nothing more influential in a child's life than the moral power of quiet example. For children to take morality seriously, they must see adults take morality seriously.

—*William J. Bennett, former secretary of education*

---

### Can You Let Your Child Make His or Her Own Decisions?

One of the opportunities that sport provides is the chance for children to acquire and practice adult behaviors. An essential part of growing up is accepting responsibility for one's own behavior and decisions. This can become a real challenge for parents because once you invite your child to make decisions, you must support and live with those decisions. As your child matures, you should offer suggestions and guidance about sports. But ultimately, within reasonable limits, you should let your child go his or her own way. All parents have ambitions for their children, but they must accept the fact that they cannot dominate their children's lives. Youth sports can offer an introduction to the major parental challenge of letting go.

### Can You Share Your Son or Daughter?

A final challenge relates to the third point in the athletic triangle, your child's coach or manager: Can you give up your child to another significant adult? Many issues can arise in your relationship with the coach, including the way in which he or she is coaching the team or relating to your child. You are putting your youngster in the charge of another adult and trusting him or her to guide the sport experience. Beyond that, you must deal with the fact that the coach may gain admiration and affection that was once yours alone. It is natural for a coach to become a very important figure in a child's life. This occurs at a time when a tendency toward independence is causing the child to move away somewhat from parents. One father described his difficulty in adjusting to his child's coach:

> I was used to being number one in Mark's life. I was the man he looked up to, the man with all the answers, the man to be like someday. Things began to change a bit when he joined the basketball league. He was placed on a team run by the most popular coach in the league, a man who had played college ball and who has a real charisma with kids. All of a sudden, all we heard at the dinner table was, "Coach said this and Coach did that." It became more and more clear that my son had a new hero, and one whom I couldn't compete with. I've thought about it a lot, and I can understand that what's happening is perfectly normal, but it's not easy to take a backseat in my child's life, even temporarily.

When parents cannot accept the entry into the child's world of a new and important adult, youngsters may suddenly find themselves in the middle of a conflict between parent and coach in which the child is subtly pressured to make a choice between the two. Like allowing your child more freedom to make decisions, sharing him or her temporarily with another valued adult (and one toward whom greater esteem seems to be shown at times) can be an important part of the process of letting go.

Sports offer your child many opportunities for personal growth and development. They also offer parent and child opportunities to interact in ways that enrich their relationship. It is our hope that this book will contribute to developing champions in sports and in life.

## A CHILD'S PLEA

Well, here it is another hockey season,
So I am writing you for just one reason.
Please don't scream or curse and yell;
Remember I'm not in the NHL.
I am only 11 years old
And can't be bought or traded or sold.
I'm not looking for hockey fame;
I just want to have fun and play the game.
Please don't make me feel as if I committed a sin,
Just because my team didn't win.
I don't want to be that great you see;
I'd rather play and just be me.
And so, in closing, I'd like to give you one tip,
Remember, the name of the game is
SPORTSMANSHIP.

—Donny Chabot, Sault Ste. Marie, Ontario

# 2

# Psychology and Young Athletes

## What Parents Can Do

The development of a human being is a truly remarkable process. In only 9 months two microscopic cells change into a fully formed human infant. Six years later the newborn has become a walking, talking first-grader ready to tackle such complex skills as reading, arithmetic, relating to others, and sports. From here, a process of rapid mental, physical, and social development advances the child into the storms and challenges of adolescence and then into such adult roles as worker, husband or wife, and parent.

> Parents have a window to the wonders of growth and development in their children.

As parents, we are excited by rapid events of evolving maturity. And, at the same time, we are saddened by the realization that we and our children can never recapture the delights of earlier ages, now preserved only in our videos, photo albums, and hearts.

Because so much of a child's time is spent in play, the functions of play have attracted the attention of scientists, medical doctors, and educators. To understand the role of sports in the life of the child, we must first consider the meaning and functions of play itself.

## PLAY AND THE DEVELOPING CHILD

Animals as well as humans engage in play activities. In animals play is a way of learning and rehearsing behaviors that are necessary for future survival. For example, baby lions stalk and pounce on objects in their play. In children, too, play has important functions during development.

From its earliest beginnings in infancy, play is a way in which children learn about the world and their place in it. Much of the first 2 years of life are spent learning about objects and events. By handling and manipulating objects in the environment, infants gain information about how to respond to the world and how it responds to them.

Between the ages of 2 and 7, children spend most of their waking hours involved in play. In their play, they take on a variety of imaginary roles. With time, they become responsive to playmates and begin to understand the effects of their actions on them. Play now becomes an important avenue for social development. Children can try out various kinds of social interactions by creating rules for games or by developing ways to cooperate, share, or compete. They can experiment with different roles and actions without actually experiencing the dangers that the real action might hold. Through make-believe play, children can test skills—such as driving a car or cooking a meal—that they might not be allowed to try in reality at that time. They can also learn new skills, such as building with blocks or mastering an electronic video game, by watching more skillful playmates.

> Play serves as a training ground for skills, knowledge, and social development.

In later childhood, play changes from the dramatic fantasy of the young child to games regulated by rules that everyone accepts. Beyond age 6, children spend a great deal of time making up exact rules, and they place strong pressure on one another to follow them. Through this process children learn that social systems are cemented together by rules and that the good of the group demands the individual's willingness to abide by the rules. This is the beginning of consideration for the rights of others. Children learn to compete, too, but within a safe world where the consequences of losing are minimized. Younger children often attach little significance to who wins or loses. In contrast to many adults, they often get their enjoyment from experiencing, not just from winning.

## ACHIEVEMENT IN SPORTS AND LIFE

The sport environment is a developmentally significant one, partly because it is an achievement setting of great relevance to the participants. For example, research has shown that children's motivation and investment are greater in sport activities than in classroom activities and interactions with their friends. Therefore, important lessons about achievement and the meaning of success and failure can be learned in athletics.

When conducted properly, youth sports can help youngsters to acquire the kinds of attitudes, values, and skills that promote achievement and success in all areas of life. When mismanaged, sports can create fear of failure, reduce enjoyment, undermine self-worth, and counter values of fair play. Which of these consequences occurs depends largely on the type of *motivational climate* that is created by coaches and parents. The motivational climate is critically important because it communicates different notions about what success is and what is required to be a "success."

Two different ways of defining success have been identified by researchers who study achievement motivation. An *ego goal orientation* is found in people who define success as winning or being better than others. They are always comparing themselves with others and don't feel successful unless they see themselves as performing better than others. Anything short of victory is failure and indicates to them that they are inferior. Carried to an extreme, the view is that "If I'm not the best, I'm the worst." For such people, the stakes are high for winning or losing, and some develop high fear of failure because, to them, failure means inferiority.

If you make winning games a life or death proposition, you're going to have problems. For one thing, you'll be dead a lot.

*—Dean Smith, Basketball Hall of Fame coach*

A second and healthier view of success is called a *mastery goal orientation*. Mastery-oriented people focus on their own effort and accomplishments instead of comparing themselves with others. In a sense, they compare themselves with themselves. They can feel success and satisfaction when they have learned something new, seen skill improvement in themselves, or given maximum effort. Even if they see themselves as less skillful than someone else, mastery-oriented people can feel competent and successful if they view themselves as doing their best to become the best they can be. In the long run, by focusing on becoming *their* best, mastery-oriented people are more likely to realize their potential and to be free of performance-destroying fear of failure that causes some athletes to "choke" under pressure.

Success is peace of mind which is a direct result of self-satisfaction in knowing you made the effort to do the best of which you are capable.

*—John Wooden, Basketball Hall of Fame player and coach*

Coach Wooden's perspective on success may be the most important reason why he deserves the title "Wizard of Westwood." He realized that everyone can be a success because success relates to the effort that one puts into realizing one's personal potential.

Ego and mastery goal orientations do not develop in a vacuum; they are acquired and reinforced by significant adults—coaches and parents. Adults create the *motivational climate* by the values they communicate, particularly about what success is, and by the behaviors they reward or punish. In an *ego-based climate*, the emphasis is on winning out over others, including both opponents and one's own teammates. It's fair to say that the following statement typifies an ego environment:

In this game, you're either a winner or a loser. Success means winning championships. Anything else is failure.

—*George Allen, Pro Football Hall of Fame coach*

In an ego-based climate, coaches often focus their attention on the most talented athletes, who have the greatest influence on winning. Effort and improvement are not emphasized as much as performance level. Rivalry among teammates may be encouraged by comparing them openly with one another. Inadequate performance or mistakes are often punished with belittlement and criticism, teaching children that mistakes are to be avoided at all costs and thereby building fear of failure. Another unfortunate outcome associated with an ego climate is the willingness to win at all costs, even if rule-breaking is required to gain the needed advantage. Obviously, this doesn't sound like a fun environment. And, in fact, athletes in such sport environments report much lower enjoyment than those in mastery environments.

In a *mastery-based climate*, the goal is to foster positive growth as an athlete and as a person. The emphasis is on effort, learning, and personal improvement—doing what it takes to be *your* best. To be sure, winning is valued, but in a mastery climate, the adults realize that winning takes care of itself if athletes are having fun, improving their skills, giving maximum effort, working together, and not being shackled with fear of failing. Mastery climates foster an atmosphere of mutual support and encouragement, and everyone, regardless of ability, is made to feel an important part of the team.

Which type of motivational climate is best for youth sports? Scientific research has provided a clear answer, and it is the same answer that has been shown in school and work settings. Mastery climates consistently have more positive effects on both achievement and on psychological factors. Seven of the beneficial effects are summarized below:

- In mastery climates, young athletes are more likely to develop intrinsic (internal) motivation for the activity, enjoying the activity for itself. In ego climates, participation is enjoyed not for itself, but instead is a means toward some other extrinsic (external) end, such as social status, recognition, or avoidance of punishment or disapproval. Whatever area of life is involved, research has shown that intrinsic motivation fosters greater enjoyment of the activity, greater persistence and personal commitment to it, and higher levels of performance. When sport participation is intrinsically motivated, young athletes enjoy it for the fun and challenge it provides and are less likely to drop out.

- Mastery climates are associated with greater sport enjoyment. In ego climates, pressures to outperform others decrease enjoyment if you're not "top dog." Not surprisingly, more kids drop out of sports from ego climates because competitive pressures decrease fun.
- Mastery climates minimize fear of failure because an emphasis on effort, persistence, and improvement is within the athlete's control. Ego climates foster fear of failure because comparisons with others (whose performance one can't control) and concerns about ability increase anxiety.
- Mastery climates tend to increase self-esteem because children are rewarded and take pride in their own improvement and effort. In ego climates, athletes may not feel good about themselves unless they outperform others, and a failure to do so may diminish feelings of self-worth.
- In mastery climates, athletes come to believe that effort is the key to success, and they value hard work and cooperation with others. In other words, they internalize John Wooden's definition of success, striving to become the best they can be. In ego climates, athletes believe that ability and "getting an edge" over others are what govern success. They are therefore more willing to cheat or use intimidation to win.
- Mastery climates, whether in sports or in school, promote faster and better skill development and higher performance than do ego climates. When athletes are enjoying themselves and focusing on effort

and improvement, and are not hampered by fear of failing, winning takes care of itself. In such cases, teams are actually more successful.

- In terms of athletes' ratings of how much fun they had and how much they liked playing for their coach, one study showed that a mastery climate was about ten times more influential than was the teams' won-lost records.

Buying into a mastery orientation means that winning becomes something different than collecting "Ws" and league championships. Let's examine this conception of what it means to be a *winner*.

## THE REAL MEANING OF WINNING

Vince Lombardi was a winner. During his years as coach of the Green Bay Packers, he created a professional football dynasty the likes of which had never been seen before. His team was the powerhouse of the NFL during the 1960s—a team driven to excellence by an intensely competitive, perfectionist leader. Lombardi's image was immortalized in the famous statement, "Winning isn't everything; it's the only thing."

If you are a sports fan or perhaps even if you are not, you have heard this famous quote. But did you know that Lombardi never actually said that? Years after his death, his son revealed that his father had been misquoted.

---

Winning isn't everything, but making the effort to win is.

—*Vince Lombardi, Pro Football Hall of Fame coach*

---

John Wooden was another winner, and so were the UCLA Bruins who played for him. During a 12-year period from 1963 through 1975, his teams won the national collegiate basketball championship ten times. Certainly to be that successful Wooden and his Bruins had to be single-mindedly focused on winning games. And yet, at least where Wooden was concerned, this was not the case. In fact, what he did communicate to his teams may be the key to their success and their ability to play well under pressure. John Wooden once told an audience of coaches:

> You cannot find a player who ever played for me at UCLA that can tell you that he ever heard me mention "winning" a basketball game. He might say I inferred a little here and there, but I never mentioned winning. Yet the last thing that I told my players just prior to tip-off, before we would go on the floor, was, "When the game is over, I want your head up, and I know of only one way for your head to be up. That's for you to know that you did your best. No one can do more. . . . You made that effort."

Yes, Lombardi and Wooden were winners. Their won-lost records speak for themselves. Yet it is interesting to note that both coaches placed an emphasis on the process of striving for excellence. Their vision went beyond a preoccupation with winning games. Instead, they demanded that their players dedicate themselves to 100 percent effort.

The common notion in sports equates success with victory—scoring more points, runs, or goals than the opponent. Yet, in a youth sport model, the measure of a person's or a team's success goes beyond records and standings. Success is a personal thing and is related to one's own standards and abilities.

In terms of the educational benefits of sport, children can learn from both winning and losing. But for this to occur, winning must be placed in a *healthy* perspective. We have therefore developed a four-part philosophy of winning designed to maximize young athletes' enjoyment of sport and their chances of receiving the positive outcomes of participation:

1. Winning isn't everything, nor is it the only thing.

Young athletes can't possibly learn from winning and losing if they think the only objective is to beat their opponents. Does this mean that children should not try to win? Definitely not! As a form of competition, sport involves a contest between opposing individuals or teams. It would be naive and unrealistic to believe that winning is not an important goal in sports. But it is not the most important objective.

To play sports without striving to win is to be a dishonest competitor. But despite this fact, it is important that we not define success only as winning. Not every child can play on a championship team or become a champion athlete. Yet every child can experience the true success that comes from trying his or her best to win. The opportunity to strive for success is the right of every young athlete.

---

The bottom line in youth sports should not be based on pressure to win. Instead, it should be on the enjoyment of competing and the opportunity to develop positive attitudes toward other people.

—*Lute Olson, Basketball Hall of Fame coach*

---

2. Failure is not the same thing as losing.

Athletes should not view losing as a sign of failure or as a threat to their personal value. They should be taught that losing a game is not a reflection of their own self-worth. In other words, when an individual or team loses a competition, it does not mean that they are worth less than if they had won. In fact, some valuable lessons can be learned from losing. Children can learn to persist in the face of obstacles and to support each other even when they do not achieve victory.

They can also learn that mistakes are not totally negative, but are important stepping-stones to achievement. Mistakes provide valuable information that is necessary for improving performance. Thomas Edison was once asked whether he was discouraged by the failure of more than three thousand experiments leading to the development of the lightbulb. Edison replied that he did not consider the experiments failures, for they had taught him three thousand ways not to create a lightbulb and each experiment had brought him closer to his goal.

3. Success does not depend on winning.

Thus, neither success nor failure need depend on the outcome of a competition or on a won-lost record. Winning and losing apply to the outcome of a competition, whereas success and failure do not. How, then, can we define success in sports?

4. Athletes should be taught that success is found in striving for victory.

The important idea is that *success is related to commitment and effort!* The only thing that athletes have complete control over is the amount of effort they give. They have only limited control over the outcome that is achieved. If we can impress on our children that they are never "losers" if they give maximum effort, we are giving them a priceless gift that will assist them in many of life's tasks. A youth soccer coach had the right idea when he told his team, "You kids are always winners when you try your best! But sometimes the other team will score more goals."

---

I have no control over results. All I can do is play to the best of my abilities. Success is me giving everything that I have.

—*Ichiro Suzuki, Major League Baseball player*

---

A major cause of athletic stress is fear of failure. When young athletes know that making mistakes or losing a competition while giving maximum effort is acceptable, a potent source of pressure is removed. Moreover, if adults apply this same standard of success to themselves, they will be less likely to define their own adequacy in terms of a won-lost record and will more likely focus on the important children's goals of participation, skill development, and fun. Parents and coaches will also be less likely to experience stress of their own when their athletes are not winning.

---

*Doing your best* is more important than *being the best*.

—*Forrest "Frosty" Westering, College Football Hall of Fame coach*

---

When winning is kept in perspective, the child comes first and winning is second. In this case, the most important sport product is not a won-lost record; it is the quality of the experience provided for the athletes.

## SPORTS AND DEVELOPMENT OF SELF-ESTEEM

During the early elementary school years, the world of the child broadens dramatically to include not only the family and playmates but a widening circle of schoolmates and adults. In this expanded environment children discover and judge their own abilities and begin to form a stable self-concept and feelings of self-worth. Academic and social experiences provide important information, as do the reactions of peers and adults in the child's life. It is during this critical period of development—the years between 6 and 12—that most children enter youth sport programs. This is why sport experiences can play such an important role in children's personal and social development.

*Self-esteem* refers to the way we *feel* about our own personal traits and abilities—as good or bad, valuable or worthless, and so on. Self-esteem strongly influences how we function in the world, and it is a product of our experiences in living.

Self-esteem underlies our view of who we are, what we are capable of, and how we can expect others to react to us.

Two types of information are particularly important with regard to self-esteem development:

- *how other people respond* to us
- *how we compare with others* in important skills and characteristics

First, from the reactions of significant people in their lives, children draw conclusions concerning how other people feel about or evaluate them. Children often have little more than the reactions of others to go on. It is no wonder that such information has such a strong influence on their sense of who they are and how worthwhile they are. Thus, a child who consistently receives attention, approval, and loving concern from parents is likely to conclude that he or she is a valued person and thereby develops high self-esteem. Such messages to the child may be very direct, as when a parent says, "You're a great kid, and I love you very much," or they may be transmitted in more subtle ways, such as approving smiles and expressions of attention and interest in the child. On the other hand, children who receive a lot of disapproval, rejection, and hostility from those who matter are likely to infer that others see them as unlovable, unworthy, and inferior. It is not surprising that such children tend to develop low self-esteem.

A second important type of information enters into development of self-esteem. At a relatively early age, children begin to compare themselves with other children. This is quite natural, for in any new or novel situation we have little basis for judging ourselves or our performance except in comparison with others. Comparison and competition begin around the age of 5 and increase throughout the elementary school years, with the peak occurring around grades four, five, and six. Through self-comparison and competition with other children, youngsters learn where they stand relative to others like them.

> The sport setting provides many opportunities for self-comparisons and reactions from others.

Psychologists who study personality place much emphasis on self-esteem because we tend to filter new information and to behave in accordance with our feelings of self-worth. We tend to accept evidence that supports our notion of ourselves, be it positive or negative, and reject or explain away evidence that is inconsistent with our self-esteem. Thus, a failure may have little impact on a child with a positive view of himself or herself, while the same failure may serve to demonstrate once again to the low-self-esteem youngster how inadequate he or she really is.

Children with low self-esteem have little confidence in their abilities. They are insecure in their relationships with others, are highly sensitive to criticism, and are easily hurt. Some try to cover up their feelings of inadequacy with an aggressive or attention-demanding front that alienates others, whereas others withdraw into a protective shell. Either response tends to result in low popularity, and this only serves to confirm a poor self-image. The low-self-esteem youngster is thus primed for entry into a failure cycle.

You can now see why sport experiences can have an important effect on a child's self-esteem development. Children typically enter the world of sports at a time in their development when they are seeking information about their abilities. The kinds of motor abilities required in sports are particularly valued by them at this stage. When children enter sports, the stage is thus set for an ability test whose outcome is potentially very important.

There are good reasons to try to succeed and to be a good athlete. Success brings feelings of mastery, competence, and self-pride; admiration and status from peers; and approval from important adults, such as parents and coaches. Inferior athletes often experience feelings of shame and inferiority, lowered respect and status among their peers, and the reactions of disappointed parents.

At the very first practice or tryout, children begin to see how they compare with their peers in this prized activity. In a very short time children can tell how proficient they are relative to their teammates and opponents.

In addition to comparing themselves with others, children also have many opportunities to observe how others are judging them. The reactions of coaches, parents, teammates, opponents, and spectators to their play are visible on many occasions. Some of these evaluations are very direct, as when others offer praise or criticism. Other reactions, although unintentionally shown, are easily picked up by a child. For example, when Brent comes to the plate with the bases loaded, his teammates, the coach, and spectators cheer and shout, "Hit a home run!" When Ryan comes up under the same circumstances, there is silence or maybe even a few groans. Or "encouragement" may take such forms as "C'mon, Ryan, try to hit the ball!" or "Don't strike out!"

In highly organized youth sport programs, formal selection and distribution procedures are used in forming teams. This includes such activities as grading youngsters during tryouts, "drafting" athletes, and even buying them with play money, all of which provide direct indications of ability.

> One young athlete was devastated when his coach paid only $25,000 in play money for him while his buddy fetched $40,000!

An even more painful experience is being cut—a most humiliating message that one doesn't measure up. Research done in Canada by sport psychologist Dr. Terry Orlick showed that nearly 75 percent of nonparticipants who didn't try out for hockey teams said they were afraid of being cut—an indication of how much children dread the message that they're not good enough.

Even children who make the team continue to receive many messages about their performance. This feedback comes from people whose opinions carry a great deal of weight because they are so important to the child. Many parents are very concerned about their children's athletic development and often have a good deal to say about performance. It is the job of another significant adult, the coach, to evaluate performance. Youngsters receive much feedback from this "expert" about their strengths, weaknesses, areas needing improvement, and progress. The coach also makes very obvious ability judgments in selecting players for particular positions, in choosing who starts and who substitutes, and in deciding the game conditions in which substitutions occur. Being allowed to play only when one's team is way ahead or hopelessly behind communicates a pretty clear message.

Athletics thus provide many opportunities for children to form judgments about their abilities. They get information by comparing themselves with others as well as by observing the reactions of others to them. All this occurs during the age period when children are beginning to form a stable conception of who they are and how they feel about themselves. If you add to this the fact that motor abilities are of central importance and highly valued at this age and that the people evaluating the child—coaches, peers, and parents—are of great importance in the child's life, is it any wonder why the experiences children have in sports can have a rather profound effect on them? This is particularly the case with children who have not established feelings of self-worth in other areas of their lives or with those whose parents value athletic abilities above all others. Finally, it is important to realize that children at this age are not yet capable of distinguishing between judgments of their abilities and judgments of their personal worth.

> At early ages, children do not necessarily see ability judgments as evaluations of only a single physical trait but may well take them as an indication of total worth.

What can parents do? To begin, adults must be sensitive to the impact that sport experiences can have on the child's self-esteem. The processes we have described—self-comparison and feedback from others—are going to occur in any situation in which children interact, but their effects can be softened and viewed more realistically if understanding adults help children place sport experiences in proper perspective. There are several things adults can do.

First and foremost you should emphasize fun, participation, and skill improvement rather than winning and losing. Most children want to play a sport because they enjoy the activity for its own sake. Adults can turn that enjoyable activity into a pressurized, competitive nightmare. Fun is no longer just playing; it's now defined as winning.

Second, adults should emphasize striving to improve skills rather than comparing oneself with others. Physical development and skill development occur at different rates in youngsters, and it is important to make this clear to children. It is particularly important that children whose skill development is lagging not view this as a permanent condition. Helping a youngster derive pleasure from his or her improvement over time and praising the self-improvement efforts of the child can create many rewarding experiences in sport—even for the athlete who never will be a star.

> Parents should emphasize fun,
> participation, and self-improvement.

Third, just as it is important that the unskilled child athlete not develop low self-worth because of his or her own sport abilities, it is important that the highly skilled athlete not acquire an inflated self-image, often expressed as arrogance and a "swelled head." Again, parents should help children to understand that despite the importance of sport to them, it is only one area of their lives. This will foster a more balanced perspective and a wider range of interests.

Finally, parents should examine the conditions of worth that they hold for their children. If your young athlete must excel to get love and approval from you, if you are sending out subtle (or not so subtle) signals of disapproval when your child fails or embarrasses you, then you need to take a hard look at your own priorities. If, on the other hand, you are able to communicate love and acceptance to your child whether he or she is a star or a benchwarmer, then a basis for positive self-esteem development exists regardless of your child's eventual achievements in sports.

Competitive experiences are an important part of life. In themselves, sports are neither good nor bad. The value of participation depends on how the competition is conducted, how the situation is interpreted, and how the outcome is understood. Properly managed, youth sports can be an important training ground for competing successfully in other areas of life and for developing positive self-esteem.

## NEEDS FOR APPROVAL AND RECOGNITION
As social beings, humans have a need to be recognized, valued, and cared about by others. From a very early age, children seem to crave attention and to do whatever is necessary to gain it. Many children with

behavior problems develop those problems because obnoxious behavior is the only way the children have of guaranteeing the attention of parents and others. Rather than being ignored, such children prefer the attention that goes along with being punished.

As children develop, they learn to satisfy their needs for recognition and approval in a variety of ways. For one thing, they find out what is praiseworthy to people who matter to them, such as parents, teachers, and peers. It doesn't take most children very long to realize that sports provide many opportunities for recognition and approval. They see how sport heroes are idolized in our culture, and they often develop their own sport heroes at a relatively early age. Further, many parents communicate very positive attitudes about sports and exhibit a great deal of interest in such activities. Finally, as we noted earlier, physical skills are among the most highly prized attributes of school-aged children.

> Approval and recognition provide powerful
> motivation for athletes at all levels.

Almost all of the positive attributes that can be developed through sport participation—achievement motivation, sportsmanship, teamwork, unselfishness—are ultimately strengthened through the approval of significant people, such as coaches, parents, and teammates. Thus, it is almost impossible to overestimate the importance of approval and recognition to the developing athlete.

As with many psychological characteristics, there are both approach and avoidance motives connected with approval. On the approach side, there is the positive desire to obtain approval and recognition from other people. The child wants approval and may be frustrated if approval is not received, but the child is not necessarily afraid of disapproval.

On the other hand, the social behavior of many people is motivated by a strong desire to avoid disapproval at all costs—a motivational state similar to fear of failure. Such people are very concerned about the evaluation of others, and they are fearful of being evaluated unfavorably. Often they automatically assume that all assessments will be negative. As a result, they may experience considerable tension and distress in social situations, and they may be highly motivated to avoid them. Where fear of disapproval is not excessive, these people enter social situations but strive to please others at all costs. They are highly conforming and hesitate to take a position of which others might disapprove. They define their own self-worth in terms of the feedback they get from other people.

For young athletes, the most important external sources of approval are coaches, parents, and teammates.

Of equally great importance, however, is the child's own approval or disapproval of himself or herself. Once children begin to set standards for their own behavior, they approve or disapprove of themselves depending on whether or not they meet these standards. Thus, children may feel badly about themselves if they do something that they know is wrong, even if their friends approve. The development of internal standards of behavior and of conditions for self-approval and self-disapproval is a sign of developing maturity in a child.

Recognizing that motivational patterns differ from child to child, we assessed the relative strength of approval motives in a research study. A psychological test was devised to measure the approval-related reasons that child athletes strive to do well in sports, and we administered the test to a large number of boys and girls of various ages. Table 2.1 shows the results of this study.

It is noteworthy that for children in both age groups, their own self-approval and disapproval were more important to them than the reactions of peers, coaches, or parents. Where parents were concerned, the younger children were more strongly oriented toward avoiding parental disapproval than toward gaining their approval, whereas the older youngsters were relatively more concerned with getting approval than

**Table 2.1. Reasons for Trying to Perform Well in Sports**

| Reason for trying to play well | Order of Importance Age | |
|---|---|---|
| | 9–11 Years | 12–14 Years |
| 1. Feeling good about how you played. | 1 | 1 |
| 2. Making sure you won't blame yourself for losing. | 2 | 2 |
| 3. Being praised by your parents for playing well. | 6 | 4 |
| 4. Making sure your parents won't be displeased with your play. | 3 | 8 |
| 5. Making your coach proud of you. | 4 | 3 |
| 6. Making sure your coach won't be displeased with you. | 5 | 6 |
| 7. Making the other kids like you more. | 8 | 7 |
| 8. Making sure the other kids don't get upset with you. | 7 | 5 |

with avoiding disapproval. It is important to note, however, that this pattern did not hold for all children, but only for the sample as a whole. For some children, the reactions of others were of utmost importance. Sometimes the primary motive was to gain approval, while other children were clearly motivated to avoid the disapproval of others.

The motives that bring children into sports and that affect their development and performance once they get there are of great importance in understanding the child athlete. These motivational factors will be covered in subsequent chapters.

## EXTRINSIC REWARDS: CAN WE DESTROY LOVE OF THE GAME?

The story is told of an elderly woman who lived in an apartment building next to a vacant lot. One afternoon as she was settling down for her daily nap, a frisky group of boys and girls appeared in the vacant lot and began a noisy soccer game. The racket was deafening and the children obviously enjoyed the game far more than the old woman did. Her only comfort was the hope that they would not come back. But, alas, the children joyfully returned the next 2 days as well.

On the third day, as the children were leaving, the woman walked down to the vacant lot and called them together. She told them that she liked to watch and listen to them play and asked them to come back and play noisily in the vacant lot the next day. If they did, she said, she would give each of them 50 cents. The children raced back the following day and had a wild game, looking occasionally up at the old woman smiling approvingly from her window. She paid each of them 50 cents and asked them to return the next day. Again the next day she paid them after their game. This time, however, she gave each child only 40 cents, explaining that she was running out of money. On the following day, they got only 15 cents each. Furthermore, she told them, she would have to reduce their payment to 10 cents the next day. The children became angry and told the woman they would not be back. It was not worth the effort, they said, to play a game for only 10 cents a day.

The old woman might very well have been a retired psychologist, for she had cleverly used external rewards, in this case money, to decrease the desire of children to play. We can assume that the children originally came to the vacant lot because of their intrinsic motivation to play soccer "for the fun of it." When money was introduced into the picture as an additional reward for playing, the children began to see themselves as playing primarily to get this extrinsic reward. Once this shift in their perception of their own motives occurred, the withdrawal of the money reduced their desire to continue playing.

Although this story is probably fictional, the principle that extrinsic rewards can undermine intrinsic motivation is not. Psychological experiments have consistently shown that this can occur in children as well as adults. In youth sports, there is the risk that children's intrinsic interest in the sport can be decreased if they begin to see their participation as a means to some material or extrinsic awards (money, trophies, ribbons, T-shirts, etc.).

If carried to an extreme, external rewards can replace intrinsic motivation as the reason for participating in sports. When the young athletes begin to see these extrinsic rewards as the reason for their participation, the removal of these rewards may result in a loss of interest in participation.

An unhappy example of exactly this effect is the case of the teenage wrestler whose father attended one of our coaching workshops. The father was very concerned because his young athlete refused to enter meets unless the winners' trophies were large enough to justify the effort.

> We are *not* suggesting that trophies and other
> extrinsic rewards be eliminated from sports.

Material awards certainly have their rightful place as a means of recognizing outstanding effort and achievement. It is important, however, that adults and children maintain a proper perspective so that tangible goods do not become the be-all and end-all of participation. It is sad indeed when children lose the capacity to enjoy athletic competition for its own sake.

### SPORTS AND CHARACTER-BUILDING

Raising our children is in large part a moral enterprise. We do our best to teach our children the difference between right and wrong. We communicate our own values to them and hope they will adopt similar values. We want them to develop positive character traits that will make them happy and contributing members of society. Our goals in this regard are shared by religious institutions, schools, youth organizations, and athletic programs. The motto of Little League Baseball—"Character, Courage, Loyalty"—exemplifies the commitment that many youth sport organizations have made to develop sportsmanship and good citizenship. In regard to this, adult leadership responsibilities go beyond teaching sport skills to include stressing the value of hard work, sportsmanship, and good citizenship.

The most important part of Little League has nothing to do with baseball.

—*H. E. Pohlman, former Washington Little League District 8 administrator*

Not everyone agrees that youth sports accomplish these goals. Critics point out that in some instances impressionable youngsters learn to swear, cheat, fight, intimidate, and hurt others. Sports provide opportunities to learn immoral values and behaviors as well as moral ones. Depending on the types of leadership provided by coaches and parents, the experiences can result in sinners as well as saints. In the final analysis, it isn't sports per se that automatically determine the worth of the activity for the child, but rather the quality of the experiences within the particular program.

Sports are an especially promising setting for learning the positive traits we lump under the term *character*. As "living laboratories," sports confront children with many challenges that await them in later life. Cooperation, competition, perseverance in the face of difficulties, concern for others, self-sacrifice, and moral behavior (sportsmanship) can all be required on any given day. Through the influence they have as important adults in children's lives, coaches and parents can teach children to respond to these challenges in desirable ways. Important lessons of life can be learned in the gymnasium and on the athletic field and court.

Many sports, particularly those that involve physical contact, require some degree of "aggressiveness" on the part of athletes. A rather fine dividing line can exist between "assertiveness" on the one hand and "aggression" on the other. Assertiveness involves using physical force to its maximum legal limit, as when a football player makes a hard tackle. Aggression, conversely, is the use of physical force in a manner that is intended to hurt an opponent. Ideally, we would like our children to be appropriately assertive, but not to intentionally try to harm others.

Unfortunately, there is evidence that sports can sometimes be a "school for violence" if parents and coaches do not teach children the

# THE YOUTH COACH AS A MORAL PHILOSOPHER

Coaches are charged with teaching young athletes not only the skills of the sport but also the value of hard work, sportsmanship, and good citizenship. To study the communication of moral values, Northwestern University sociologist Dr. Gary Fine and his colleagues observed baseball coaches over a 3-year period. Among the themes the coaches stressed were effort, sportsmanship, and teamwork. Here are some examples of their comments:

Coach during a preseason practice session:

Your goal for the year is to be a winner. That doesn't mean winning every game. Sometimes you'll be up against teams that are better than you. It does mean to give everything you've got. If you give everything that you've got, you're a winner in my book. The only one who cares is the Man that made you, and He made both teams—both winners and losers. Give everything you've got!

Coach after his team loses a game 5–1:

You guys are sleeping out there. If you have no pride in yourself, I don't want to coach you. . . . In other games, even in games in which you guys won, there was a lack of hustle. . . . I won't quit on you. Don't quit on me.

Coach when his team was ahead 8–0:

Guys, you've got a big lead. I don't want any horsing around out there. I want you to be good sports.

Coach after a come-from-behind victory:

Isn't that great to come back and win? It was a team effort. Everybody contributed and played well.

difference between assertiveness and aggression. A study of Canadian minor hockey players by Dr. Michael Smith of York University indicated that most of the players had learned illegal and violent techniques by watching and playing hockey. Among players who had learned illegal tactics, more than 60 percent reported using the tactics themselves during the season. Moreover, even at the 9- and 10-year-old level, nearly 60 percent of the children approved of fighting, even though it is against the rules. Among older players, this increased to 84 percent. Clearly, adults must be sensitive to the potential that certain "contact" sports have for teaching and rewarding aggression so that they can emphasize the importance of hard but fair play.

---

I went to a fight the other night, and a hockey match broke out!

—*Rodney Dangerfield, comedian/actor*

---

In our attempts to teach children desirable attitudes and behaviors, it is important that we explain to them the principles or reasons behind desired actions. For example, rather than threatening to punish athletes for heckling opponents, a coach might help his athletes understand the golden rule—"Do unto others as you would have them do unto you"— by asking them to consider what it would be like to be the victims of heckling. This procedure encourages athletes to develop empathy for their opponents. The ability to place oneself in the role of another person is essential to the development of morality. Understanding and applying this golden rule can thus lead children to internalize the concept of sportsmanship and consideration for others.

> Sport experiences are full of valuable lessons
> for children and can be an important training ground
> for moral and social development.

Youngsters learn moral behavior not only through verbal explanations, rewards, and punishments but also by observing how other people behave. They imitate their parents and peers, and they model themselves after their heroes. Because coaches are often highly admired and very important in the child's life, they are especially likely to serve as models. Without realizing it, coaches can behave in ways that teach either morality or immorality. For example, by trying to get a "competitive edge" by stretching the rules, coaches can easily give children the impression that cheating is not really wrong unless it is detected, and then only to the extent that it hurts the chances of winning. When coaches bend the rules in order to obtain a victory, children may conclude that the end justifies the means. Likewise, coaches who display hostility toward officials and contempt for the other team communicate the notion that such behaviors are appropriate and desirable. Even when coaches and parents preach correct values, it is essential that they themselves behave in accordance with them. Psychological experiments with children have repeatedly shown that when adults' actions are inconsistent with their words, it is the actions (not the words) that influence children's behavior. Actions do indeed speak louder than words.

> In teaching moral values, what we do
> is as important as what we say.

Critics of youth sports sometimes attack the competitive aspect of sports as inconsistent with the development of morality and concern for others. Some, however, dispute this position, arguing that moral development is actually furthered when moral decisions come into conflict with winning. In other words, noteworthy acts of sportsmanship often involve situations in which conduct governed by a moral principle (for example, one should not cheat) is chosen instead of victory. When a youngster makes a decision to do the right thing rather than unfairly pursue an opportunity to win, we have a true demonstration of moral growth. Coaches and parents are in a position to further such growth.

What, then, is the verdict on sports as a means of building character? At this point we are unable to give a definite answer, for sports are simply one aspect of the complexity of children's lives. Scientific evidence is inconclusive, although positive differences in academic achievement and personality traits are sometimes found when groups of child athletes are compared with nonathletes. Moreover, a lower incidence of juvenile delinquency has consistently been found in child athletes. The difficulty or shortcoming is proving that these differences are *caused* by sport participation. Perhaps brighter and better-adjusted children are more likely to be attracted to sports, and that's why participation is related to these attributes. There is no denying, however, that sports are capable of furthering the character development of children if adults are able to appropriately structure sport experiences for them.

3

# Physical Development
## *Young Athletes' Bodies and Performance*

An athlete's body greatly affects his or her performance potential and has much to do with the enjoyment and satisfaction that comes from training and competition. What are the features of body structure that affect sport performance? Height is an obviously important characteristic. There is always one 5-foot, 8-inch guard in a high school basketball tournament, but the 6-foot, 6-inch player has a better chance of excelling. Weight is another aspect of body size that determines potential success. The 200-pound football player has a distinct playing advantage over an opponent who weighs only two-thirds as much.

Body build, or physique, must also be considered. The three major body types (somatotypes) are described as follows:

- Endomorphs are characterized by a soft roundness throughout the body, with a tendency toward fatness.
- Mesomorphs are muscular individuals with large, prominent bones.
- Ectomorphs have thin body segments and relatively poor muscle development.

Successful athletes in a particular sport tend to have
similar body builds, and their physiques are compatible
with the requirements of the activity.

Being a mesomorph or an ectomorph will have a lot to do with whether an individual must be satisfied with recreation jogging or will enjoy working his or her long, thin legs in competitive distance races. But having a certain body type does not guarantee success or failure. The outcome is not absolute. With this in mind you can help your child select sports that are in harmony with his or her body build. This will give your child a better chance to achieve higher levels of performance.

In addition to body size and build, athletic performance is influenced by body composition—the relative amounts of bone, muscle, and fat that make up body mass. The role of muscle in moving the body and generating force is of prime importance. Quite simply, the more strength and power that an athlete has, the greater his or her advantage will be. On the other hand, fatty tissue represents excess baggage and is a performance-inhibitor. Fatness reduces speed, limits endurance, and, in some sports, increases the risk of injury. In almost all sports, with the exception of sumo wrestling perhaps, elite athletes strive to be trim and muscular, with healthy minimal levels of body fat.

Body structure and function are important in
determining how satisfying and enjoyable sports can be.

The physical characteristics that determine sport performance are constantly changing during the growing years of childhood and adolescence. Knowing something about the nature and extent of normal growth will help answer crucial questions about *what sport for what child at what age*. Moreover, such information makes it possible to project realistic expectations of sport performance on our children and to direct training programs that their changing bodies will respond to. As boys and girls move through the exciting stages of growing up in sport, some appreciation of the ever-changing body can make the experience the satisfying one it should be.

## FACTORS THAT INFLUENCE BODY CHARACTERISTICS

No two human bodies are exactly the same, not even identical twins. Body size, shape, and composition, as well as the body's million physiological characteristics, are unique to each individual. These physical traits are influenced by age and sex, along with a host of internal and external (environmental) factors. For example, the endocrine glands secrete hormones directly into the bloodstream. Hormones are basically regulators of body functions, and they play an important role in physical growth and sexual maturation. With respect to environmental forces, body structure and function depend on how adequate nutrition has been, how free from disease the body has been, and how physically active one has been.

Most importantly, body characteristics are determined by genetics. Certainly, we know that parent height is a prime determinant of offspring height. Hereditary influences on body structure and its many functions are so important in determining the potential for athletic performance that it is often said that great athletes are born, not made. The significance of one's genetic endowment cannot be denied.

Aside from the size, shape, and makeup of the body, several ways in which body functions respond to exercise and training are important contributors to athletic performance. As with the body's structure, these abilities to respond to training are in large part determined by genetic characteristics. They include: (a) the potential for developing outstanding muscle strength, (b) the capability of producing muscle energy efficiently, and (c) the capability of increasing the body's metabolism to a very high level to meet the demands of vigorous exercise. Quick reaction and speed of movement are also important to the athlete. These traits are greatly influenced by heredity.

> If someone wishes to develop the body of an elite athlete
> and the potential to respond ideally to a sport training program,
> the individual should select his or her parents with great care.

We've emphasized that hereditary factors are critical in determining which children can look forward to being outstanding, and perhaps even elite, athletes. However, the effects of genetics are never absolute because genes do not operate in isolation. We cannot undervalue the influence of the environments in which we live—natural, social, and athletic. During childhood and adolescence, regular exercise is among the many environmental factors essential to achieving full potential for growth. Moderate physical stress from the muscle activities found in most sports is generally a positive force on bone growth. But training programs for young athletes have virtually no growth-promoting effect on their height. Dramatic exercise effects do, however, occur in muscle and adipose (fat) tissue. Following the start of adolescence in males, the increase in muscle mass is directly related to the intensity and duration of training programs. And, of course, the loss of fatty tissue from exercise is a desirable effect of sport participation.

On the side of caution, relatively little is known about the limits beyond which strenuous physical activity can be harmful to a young athlete's growth. Unfortunately, there is no exact guide for determining how much activity is optimal. The issue includes consideration of the maturation level of the child, the frequency and duration of the activity (the problem of energy depletion), and the adequacy of nutrition (normal caloric intake). The most reasonable approach is to rely on the child's own tolerance. The young athlete will generally know when his or her limit has been reached.

A related and equally important issue concerns the exercise tolerance of healthy children. Do endurance sports place *excessive* demands on the hearts of young athletes? No. This is a popular myth. There is increasing evidence that the growing child's heart responds favorably to the normal levels of physical exertion in such sports.

Children's exercise tolerance is greater than believed in the past.

The key to safely handling the demands of heavy exercise resides in the health of the child. This points to the need for careful medical screening, which includes probing for a family history of cardiac problems and any early cardiovascular difficulties. Also, in protecting the wellness of child athletes, parents cannot ignore the importance of appropriate endurance-training procedures that are supervised by competent coaches.

## PATTERNS OF PHYSICAL GROWTH

There is an abundance of information concerning the growth of American children. Growth can be looked at merely as heights or weights for given ages, as seen in figure 3.1. These curves indicate a child's growth status or the size attained at a particular age.

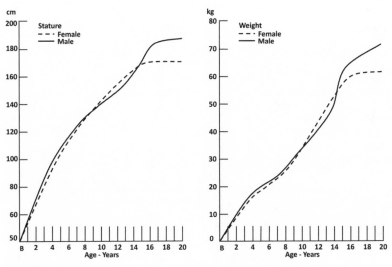

FIGURE 3.1
Typical growth curve in height and weight for boys and girls. For height, 2.54 cm = 1 inch; for weight, 1 kg = 2.2 pounds.

It is interesting to look at the increases in height and weight that occur during a given period of time. The velocity curves shown in figure 3.2 illustrate the rate of growth, that is, centimeters or kilograms gained per year. We can see that the most rapid period of growth occurs immediately after birth, and then the growth rate slows to a modest, steady process during childhood. This is followed by an adolescent growth spurt and then by deceleration until growth finally stops. There is little difference in the relative growth rates of boys and girls during childhood. However, as shown in figure 3.1, during childhood years, boys are slightly taller and heavier than girls of the same age. This difference is a relatively minor one and of no real practical significance for sport performance.

When girls experience the rapid growth spurt that occurs between the ages of 10.5 and 13, they become taller than boys. During pubescence, tall girls will be taller than tall boys, and all girls will be taller than the shortest 3 to 5 percent of boys. This is a temporary situation that changes when boys begin to experience their adolescent growth spurt

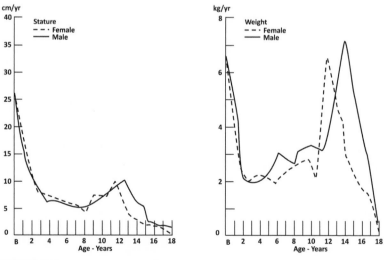

FIGURE 3.2
Velocity curves showing rates of increase in height and weight.

in height some 2 years after girls have experienced their peak velocity in gaining height.

> Girls are nearer their final body size at any age because they mature at a faster rate than boys.

Prior to adolescence, sex differences in body composition are minor. However, boys do have slightly more bone and muscle tissue and less fat than girls. Following the period of maximum gain in height that occurs in early adolescence (about age 12 to 13 for girls and 14 to 15 for boys), there is a period of maximum gain in weight. In girls, this is due primarily to a large increase in body fat, with a relatively small increase in muscle tissue. In boys, the rapid gain in body weight that follows a rapid gain in height is due primarily to a decrease in relative body fatness and a striking increase in muscle mass. Consequently, postadolescent girls have only about two-thirds as much muscle as males, and young adult females have almost twice the amount of body fat as males.

Because boys, on the average, begin their rapid gain in height at the age of 12.5, they have about 2 more years of preadolescent growth than girls have. During this 2-year period, they continue to grow, and at age 14 or 15, they are about 4 inches taller than girls were when they began their rapid growth. In the immediate preadolescent period, boys' legs grow much faster than their trunks. Thus, the longer period of preadolescent growth for males is responsible for the fact that legs of adult males are longer than those of females.

> All boys and girls experience an adolescent growth spurt.

The age at which the adolescent growth spurt begins varies widely from one individual to another. The variation is so great in a sample of normal males, for example, that some boys may have their most rapid growth as early as their twelfth birthday, whereas others will not have this growth experience until they are nearly 16. These slower-maturing boys will not have their muscle growth and rapid gain in body weight until more than 14 months later, at 17 or 18 years of age. A very normal, but slowly maturing young male will have completed high school before he is physically equipped to compete in many sports requiring large size, strength, and a mature skeleton.

The differences in age at which adolescent growth and physical development occur are most evident during junior high school or middle school, or at 12 to 15 years of age. Normal boys can vary as much as 15 inches in height, 90 pounds in weight, and 5 years in maturation status, that is, biological age. (Biological age is commonly determined by an X-ray examination of skeletal maturation.) Most youth sport programs match competitors on the basis of their calendar age. Therefore, large numbers of boys, who do not experience their growth and maturation close to the average, risk some very significant problems. This is true for both the slow later maturer and the advanced early maturer. We will discuss these specific concerns later in the chapter.

## CHANGES IN PHYSICAL ABILITIES DURING CHILDHOOD AND ADOLESCENCE

During the childhood years, as boys and girls grow—resulting in longer levers and increased muscle tissue—both have the potential to increase their strength. Boys and girls show similar increased ability to perform motor skills prior to puberty. However, in general, boys are eventually able to develop greater strength and thus surpass girls in the performance of most sport-related skills.

During adolescence, males show a steady increase in performance and endurance that extends into early adulthood. The same is not true for girls. There has been a tendency for girls' performance to reach a plateau around the time of puberty (approximately 13 years of age) and decline thereafter. Because of physical changes that accompany adolescence, such as increases in fat, females are placed at somewhat of a disadvantage for motor performance. But the leveling off and subsequent decline in girls' performance and endurance are more related to sociocultural factors than to biological changes.

> For adolescent females, decreased motivation and increased
> sedentary habits are major causes of lowered performance.

Like other components of motor skill, strength shows a steady increase during childhood, with boys being slightly stronger than girls. Boys continue to improve during adolescence, whereas girls' strength scores level off and then tend to decrease. Boys experience a delay, on the average, of at least 14 months between the period of the most rapid gain in height and the most rapid gain in muscle weight. The adolescent male who is nearing the completion of his rapid gain in height will have little muscle tissue and strength potential for the next year or two. He must await the development of muscles to go along with his newly acquired taller body. Thus, the adolescent male is not as strong as his stature might suggest.

This lag in strength was apparent in a 7-foot, 2-inch college basketball freshman who had not yet begun his muscle maturation and weight gain. At 7-2 he weighed only 172 pounds. When he suffered a muscle strain, his coach remarked, "This is good news and bad news. The bad news is that he is going to miss practice for several days. The good news is that now we know he has a muscle!"

For many years, it was believed that preadolescents could not significantly improve their strength through weight training. This was attributed to insufficient amounts of muscle-building hormones (androgens) in the bloodstream prior to puberty. However, research has well documented that preadolescent boys and girls can indeed achieve measurable increases in strength. In studies conducted over 8 to 14 weeks of training with hydraulic resistance equipment, weight machines, and free weights, strength-trained subjects increased strength by 22 to 74 percent in various tests, compared with 3 to 14 percent for nonstrength-trained subjects. Such increases before puberty are more the result of neuromuscular adaptation (motor learning) than muscular adaptation (hypertrophy). In other words, prepubescent youngsters may gain strength by learning to use their muscles more effectively through practice.

> Weight training should not occur without
> highly competent adult supervision.

Because the increase in weight of the adolescent female is due primarily to a gain in fat (and, to only a small extent, to a gain in muscle), her potential for strength development via exercise is much less than the male's. In young adult women, weight training has been shown to produce significant gains in strength, but in the absence of significant amounts of male hormones (androgens), the female will experience less marked gains in the size and mass of muscles.

## SHOULD BOYS AND GIRLS COMPETE AGAINST EACH OTHER?

We have pointed out that during childhood, only very slight sex differences in body structure and motor performance are present. On a purely physical basis, there is no reason why prepubescent boys and girls should not be on the same teams competing with and against each other. The levels of performance and the chances for causing or sustaining injury related to size and strength do not differ significantly between the two sexes during childhood.

> After puberty, girls should have separate
> but equal opportunities for sport participation.

The situation changes drastically during adolescence. As boys gain more in height, weight, muscle mass, and strength, it is not possible for girls to *fairly* and *safely* compete against them in most sports. After age 11, boys and girls should have their own competitive opportunities in those sports in which strength and body size are determinants of proficiency and injury risk.

## THE GROWING AND MATURING SKELETON

The body skeleton is obviously involved in the normal growth of children. In adolescents, the skeleton first grows in size and length, after which it gains in density and strength. As mentioned earlier, the principal sites of growth before the start of rapid adolescent growth are in the legs and arms. During the adolescent growth spurt, the trunk grows most rapidly. The long bones of the arms and legs increase their length by the activity of specialized cells located in a so-called growth plate at either end of the shaft of long bones.

Because it is composed of cartilage (soft tissue), the growth plate is structurally the weakest part of the bone. It is weaker than any point in the shaft of the bone and actually weaker than the ligaments that align the neighboring joints. Additionally, the growth plate is weakest during periods of most rapid growth. Injury to this area of the bone can destroy those cells responsible for the future growth of the long bone. During the period of the most rapid gain in height (on the average, ages 14 to 15 in boys and 12 to 13 in girls), severe injury to the ends of long bones can threaten the growth plate. Growth arrest (stoppage) and a shortened leg could result in lifelong crippling if a long bone of the leg is involved.

> The growth plate of the young athlete is vulnerable to injury.

Fortunately, growth-plate injuries are not common in sports. But the threat of a growth-plate injury might temporarily direct early adolescents away from participation in collision sports, such as football and wrestling, where severe blows to a leg or arm may be encountered. As the skeleton matures, the bones become denser, stronger, and more able to withstand the trauma of hard use in intensive training. Finally, as growth nears completion in later adolescence, the growth plate ceases its function, fuses firmly with the shaft of the long bone, and is no longer the site of vulnerability that it was during early adolescence.

## SPORT PARTICIPATION AND PHYSICAL MATURITY

We have mentioned that body structure and a variety of basic functions that relate to athletic performance undergo striking change during the early years of adolescence. And there is great variation in the age at which individuals experience these changes. Therefore, the age at which children (boys in particular) are physically ready for many types of sports will also vary greatly. Youth sport programs present the early adolescent (middle school– or junior high–aged person) with opportunities for highly competitive sports. It thus becomes important to identify late-maturing and early-maturing individuals if they are to be directed into appropriate sport experiences. The late maturer will have increased risk of injury, with his undeveloped muscles and immature skeleton. Additionally, playing with and competing against larger, stronger, and more mature boys, the late maturer will be a less-skilled athlete. He is a prime candidate to drop out at the earliest opportunity.

The considerable variation in the onset of physical development during adolescence raises questions about the appropriateness of collision sports for middle school and junior high school boys. After one junior high football game, 22 players were weighed. They varied in weight from 84 to 212 pounds. Although the players' physical maturity was not technically assessed, the range of maturity seemed also to be extremely varied—as much as four or five years' variation in skeletal maturity. Unless rather elaborate steps are taken to match competitors on the basis of maturity and size in football, wrestling, and ice hockey, it is a difficult challenge to justify these sports for middle and junior high school programs.

### The Early Maturer

The early-maturing individual is bigger, stronger, and quicker; acquires sport skills faster; and has more endurance potential than his peers. Thus, the early-maturing boy can be expected to be a star grade school and junior high school athlete.

That early-maturing boys excel in several juvenile athletic programs has been well documented. In football and track-and-field events, early maturity has been shown to be a prime determinant of proficiency. Players at the Little League World Series have been studied using bone-age X-rays to document their maturation status. In one report, 71 percent of these 12-year-olds had advanced bone ages. Those with the most advanced bone age were pitchers, first basemen, left fielders, and those who batted fourth (cleanup) in the batting order. In one World Series, the winning pitcher in the championship game was a very mature 5-foot, 8-inch, 174-pound 12-year-old.

> **The difference in ability level of young athletes is often a result of different maturity levels.**

A major problem is that the early maturer enjoys outstanding sport success during elementary, middle, and early junior high school simply because of the physical advantages he has over his teammates and opponents. With the elaborate sport programs available in most communities, the 8- to 12-year-old can readily become a true sports star. That winning Little League pitcher mentioned above was flown to New York from the West Coast to appear on a national prime-time television show, and he was given a page and a half write-up in *Sports Illustrated*. A local television commentator even suggested that the junior high school where he had just started seventh grade be named after him. Pretty heady stuff for a 12-year-old.

The sport success of an early-maturing boy can lead to a full-time commitment to one or more sports at a very early age. Sport achievements may eliminate the desire for accomplishment in other areas, such as schoolwork or the arts, or an interest in exploring other sports. Positive reinforcements come from coaches, teammates, and most particularly parents, who sometimes begin to think of their star athlete in terms of outstanding high school performances, college scholarships, and perhaps even a high-salaried career in professional sports.

The world can fall apart for this youngster and his family about high school time, when as a sophomore he lines up against some juniors and seniors who possess his same maturity. Having lost the advantage of his early development, the young man is now less than an outstanding athlete. As all of his former grade school teammates and opponents catch up to him in maturity and as other athletes begin to do outstanding things, the grade school star may find only an uncomfortable place on the bench. Unable to understand the true reason that the star no longer outshines others, insensitive coaches and even parents may accuse him of "dogging it." The young man has lost the limelight of sport success on which his self-esteem was built. He is left with no other interests or talents because of his early all-consuming commitment to the sport, and he is keenly aware of the great disappointment he is to his parents. At 16 or 17, an age of considerable vulnerability to a number of disturbing antisocial alternatives, he is a depressed has-been.

> The potential problems of early-maturing athletes
> are fairly easy to avoid.

The answer, of course, is to prevent the problems from occurring. This can be done by first recognizing the signs of early maturity. The early maturer will probably be the son of a father who likewise was an early maturer, and he will experience growth changes and sexual maturation well ahead of "normal" schedule. Once identified as an individual who is maturing more rapidly than usual, he should have the opportunity to participate in sports with individuals who are of similar maturity, not the same calendar age. The early-maturing star basketball player of junior high school should have a chance to work out with the high school junior varsity. Matches can be arranged for the 12-year-old tennis star with some 16-year-old members at the tennis club. Early-maturing boys need to know how really good they are if they are to keep their athletic performances and potentials in proper perspective.

### The Late Maturer

With sport successes so closely related to maturity, it isn't difficult to imagine the problems of the late-maturing boy—especially for parents who were late maturers themselves. Many, but certainly not all, late maturers will be small in stature for their age. They will have less strength, endurance, and skeletal maturity and lower motor skills than their average peers. These boys are going to be handicapped in many sports where size, strength, and endurance determine the outcome; and in some situations, they will be at undue risk for injury.

The late-maturing individual will often be recognized as such in his elementary school years. And, as true for the early maturer, a father's own maturation experience can be an indicator of the maturation rate to be expected of the son. If early sport participation is important for the late maturer, he should be directed to sports that are not primarily dependent on size and strength for proficiency, such as racket sports, diving, and some track events. He may not become state champion, but he may achieve levels of accomplishment sufficient to earn him a satisfying place in the sport scene.

It is most important that late-maturing boys know the normal sequence of changes that occur during adolescence so that they know where they are in the maturation process, where they are going, and when they get there. With this insight, they will know when sports can be rewarding, when a vigorous training program can be effective, and when they can be sufficiently competitive on the field or court. It is possible at ages 14 to 16 to avoid a devastating negative sport experience due to delayed maturity. The late maturer doesn't have to suffer consistent setbacks and be turned off to sports and their benefits.

> Late-maturing youngsters need understanding
> and special attention from parents and coaches.

Parents and coaches should know the implications of delayed adolescent development in these boys, and they should develop their expectations accordingly. Moderate training for strength and endurance during the first two years of high school should be accompanied by large doses of encouragement on the court or field and at home. Properly managed, the late maturer can be a budding sport star by the senior year of high school. Being constantly yelled at by a coach or put down by a disappointed parent can produce a demoralized dropout at an age when dropping out can have serious ramifications.

## THE BODY OF TODAY'S YOUNG ATHLETE

Those responsible for sport programs for children and youth must recognize that athletes are a different population from those of a generation or two ago. Athletes today are bigger and stronger at younger ages. Particularly at the junior and senior high school levels, the "new model" athletes not only perform better, they demand a higher degree of sophistication and concern in dealing with their protective equipment, training facilities, coaching, refereeing, and even rule changes.

> The young athlete's body is a prime determinant of proficiency and satisfaction in sports.

Since physical features are constantly changing during childhood and adolescence, sport programs and expectations must be adjusted according to these developmental changes. Prior to the age of 12 or 13, youth sports should be for learning the fundamental skills of different sports and experiencing a variety of opportunities. During those rapidly changing years from 12 to 16, with their tremendous variation in adolescent body changes, more attention should be paid to the proper matching of competitors. Young athletes should ideally be of a similar maturational level regardless of their calendar ages. Sports provide a critical opportunity to acquire much-needed confidence in oneself and in one's newly developed body. The adolescent should not be denied this opportunity or have a negative experience because of inappropriate matching or the unrealistic performance expectations of parents and coaches.

# 4

# Choosing a Sport Program

## A First Step to a Good Experience

Sara had a lot of potential. She was strong and well coordinated and had outstanding balance. She also had an intense competitive spirit and a genuine interest in gymnastics. But that's all gone now.

Because of Sara's interest in gymnastics, her parents enrolled her in an athletic club near her home. Although the facility was excellent, the program left a lot to be desired from both a medical and psychological point of view. The coach was a hard-driving man who demanded total dedication from youngsters. "Dedication" was instilled by threats that those who did not develop fast enough would not be entered in meets. Daily practices were pressured and exhausting. There was no time for friends or other activities. Like some of the other gymnasts, Sara was put on a highly restrictive diet without medical consultation. At one point, the coach suggested that she take illegal steroids to increase her strength. His constant prodding to attempt more dangerous routines resulted in repeated injuries. After a year in the club, Sara completely burned out. She dropped out of gymnastics and vowed never to have anything to do with the sport again.

Cody's story is different. His mother and father were divorced when he was very young. Because his mother was forced to work, he had little parental guidance. As early as the second grade, Cody began to have conduct problems in school. A few years later, he became involved with a youth gang and ended up under arrest for shoplifting. He seemed well on his way to a life of delinquency. Cody's life turned around when his mother enrolled him in the local YMCA, where he came under the influence of a supervisor who steered him into the Youth Basketball Association league. Here Cody found a constructive outlet for his energies, and he developed a sense of belonging. His mother's work schedule allowed her to attend his games, and he felt great pride in being part of the team. His conduct problems in school disappeared, and he began to apply himself to his schoolwork just as he had to basketball.

Cody's story has a happy ending, whereas Sara's is tragic. One youngster found fulfillment in a sport program. The other was turned off as a result of a bad experience. Their stories illustrate the importance of selecting a good program.

Many children play sports more or less through chance. They enter a program as a result of doing what their friends are doing; or it might be a matter of practical factors, such as location and availability. In such cases, parents typically know relatively little about a program, its philosophy, or the nature of the leadership provided.

To ensure that participation occurs in high-quality programs, there is much to be said for parental involvement and guidance in the selection process. Youngsters can't be expected to critically evaluate a particular sport program. They need the assistance of their parents. If an appropriate program is selected, many unnecessary difficulties and problems can be avoided. Therefore, we strongly recommend that you take the time and effort to arrive at a well-informed choice.

## YOUR RESPONSIBILITY AS A PARENT

Parents have both the right and the responsibility to inquire about *all* activities that their children are involved in, including sports. You should take this responsibility seriously, probing into the nature and the quality of specific sport programs. By so doing, you are not being overly protective or showing a lack of confidence in a program. Rather, you are fulfilling a child-rearing obligation to oversee the welfare of your loved one.

> It is important that you gather the information necessary
> to make the right decision for you and for your child.

Inquiries by parents, if made appropriately, should be welcomed by sport-program directors and coaches. They, like you, should have as their major concern the welfare of your child. If your inquiries are not welcomed or even responded to, you have cause for concern about the program.

## DECIDING TOGETHER

Selection of a program should be a joint decision of parent and child. Although you have the final say in the matter, it is important to involve your child in the decision-making process, taking into account very seriously what your child wants to get out of the sport experience. It is a mistake for parents to assume that they know what a child wants without asking him or her. A parent whose goal is for the youngster to excel as an athlete might choose a different program than one who takes into account simply the child's desire to participate with his or her friends. A direct discussion in which you share your own experiences and opinions with your youngster rather than force them on him or her is the best approach.

> Because youth sports are run by human beings,
> you should not expect to find a fault-free program.

Most programs have certain flaws, but this does not mean that the entire experience will be a bad one for your child. If you make a commitment to work with—not against—a program, you may be able to help correct any shortcomings.

## HOW EARLY SHOULD CHILDREN PARTICIPATE?

This is not an easy question to answer, for children differ a great deal in their maturity, their aspirations, and their abilities. For this reason it is impossible to recommend a specific age for participation of all children in all sports. In the final analysis it depends on your child's characteristics, the sport in question, and the nature of the program. Children should not be rushed into organized athletics; they need time to enjoy free play with their friends, for much development occurs in such play. Certainly one important indicator of readiness is the child's own expression of interest in participating. But parents and coaches must fall back on common sense to make a decision in a particular case.

> The best guide is to know the child, the sport, and the program.

Based on available scientific and medical evidence, and taking into account individual differences in physical and psychological readiness to compete, we recommend the following age guidelines:

- Noncontact sports (baseball, swimming, track, tennis): 6 or 7 years
- Contact sports (soccer, basketball, wrestling): 8 to 10 years
- Collision sports (tackle football, hockey): 10 to 12 years

In reality, children begin to play sports at younger ages than recommended above. However, many "start-up"-type programs are appropriately modified to correspond with the developmental readiness of the participants. For example, T-ball and mini-mod soccer are excellent for introducing children to the fundamental concepts and basic skills of baseball and soccer.

### WHICH SPORTS SHOULD YOUR CHILD PLAY?

Again, there is no simple answer to this question. Along with focusing on your youngster's interests, there are additional factors to be taken into account. Such factors as safety, the benefits of individual versus team sports, and the season of the year may all influence decisions. You may be perfectly happy to have your child play outdoor soccer during warm months, but have health concerns about the same sport during cold winter months.

Parents often inquire about the benefits of individual versus team sports. Unfortunately, there is no reliable scientific research to help guide decisions. However, we can make some broad and general comparisons. On the whole, team sports offer more opportunities for learning social skills and making friends. There is also more need for cooperation and a willingness to sacrifice personal interests for the good of the team. More opportunities exist in team sports to find a niche suited to personal skills and limitations. For example, a youngster with a poor throwing arm can play first base in baseball, and a big youngster with a poor shooting touch can become a rebounding terror in basketball. In contrast, athletes in individual sports, such as tennis, need to be able to master all the skills of the sport. Finally, it is often the case that team sports generate more camaraderie, or "we" feelings, than do individual sports. Many youngsters are attracted to the sense of belonging that exists in team sports.

Individual sports generally require more self-sufficiency. The athlete cannot rely on anyone else to take up the slack. Competition takes the form of one-on-one duels, and success or failure is shouldered solely by the individual. There is also less of the social support that is provided by teammates in team sports. This can foster a strong sense of personal responsibility and independence. Because of these factors, individual sports tend to be more intensely competitive at a personal level and often demand more in the way of "mental toughness." Also, more personal dedication is often required of the athlete in training.

---

**Boxing should be banned, forbidden, and eliminated forever as a sport for children.**

—*Dr. Rainer Martens, sport psychologist and youth sport authority*

---

We feel that almost all sports have something to offer children. However, we do have major reservations about boxing. Boxing is the only sport in which the goal is to harm another person. Reports of 12-year-old boxers who have registered strings of knockouts are chilling reminders of the basic brutality of the sport. Although we acknowledge the fact that some underprivileged youths have found social and economic salvation through boxing, we do not believe that boxing in itself offers any benefits that cannot be achieved through other less dangerous sports.

### HOW MANY SPORTS SHOULD YOUR CHILD PLAY?

No matter how enjoyable or fulfilling sport participation is, it does take time and divert attention from other activities. For most children, one sport at a time is plenty during the school year. The time and energy demands on both children and their parents need to be kept at a reasonable level.

During the summer months multiple-sport participation seems more reasonable. A child may have enough time and energy to be involved in several sports, such as baseball, tennis, and swimming.

> Sometimes the best decision is not to participate.

Participation in sports, although desirable, is not necessarily for everyone. Parents should not feel that their child must be on a team or involved in a sport. For those children who wish to direct their energies in other ways, the best program may be no program. Many parents become unnecessarily alarmed if their child does not show an interest in sports. They think that a child who would rather do other things must somehow be abnormal. Forcing a child into sports against his or her will can be a big mistake. Sometimes the wisest decision is to encourage the child to move into other activities that may be more suited to his or her interests and abilities, at least until an interest in sports develops.

### SOURCES OF INFORMATION AND HOW TO GET IT

Many programs have preseason meetings to provide parents with information and to answer their questions. Such meetings can also serve as forums for parents to give input regarding concerns, opinions, and suggestions. When you attend a meeting of this kind, look for openness on the part of administrators. They should show a willingness to exchange information with the intent of promoting greater understanding and cooperation. If a program does not have such a meeting, you might suggest it to the administrator and perhaps volunteer to assist in its organization.

> A preseason sport orientation meeting
> is a good investment for everyone.

If a preseason meeting is not scheduled for parents, you may have to obtain information directly from the program administrators or coaches. Make up a list of questions and concerns before speaking with them. In dealing with program leaders, remember that they are devoting their time and effort for the benefit of youngsters who participate in their program. They deserve courtesy and your respect!

Another very useful source of information about a program is parents of athletes who have been through it. They can provide firsthand and candid feedback concerning the merits and shortcomings of the program. As consumers of the program, they may be in the best position to evaluate it for you.

### SOME IMPORTANT CONSIDERATIONS IN DECIDING ON A PROGRAM

Eventually the decision will come down to whether or not to join a particular program. Sometimes you might be choosing among several alternatives, such as the church-sponsored basketball league, the one sponsored by your local recreation department, or the one at the junior high. At other times, there may be only one program available, and your decision will be based on whether it meets your child's needs and whether the costs or possible physical risks involved are balanced by the benefits. In either of these cases, there are some key points about sport programs that you should keep in mind to help guide your decision.

**Organization and Administration**

The success of any program depends on how it is run and who is running it. You should make it a point to find out whether the program is administered by one person or by a board of directors (which is likely to include a wider range of viewpoints and representation). Of crucial importance is the extent to which you as a parent can have an influence on decisions that will affect your child.

> Potential problems can occur when a program is run by a small clique that is not open to input from parents.

Programs also vary in how much information they give parents about policies and procedures. Parents should be given an account of how revenues are spent to benefit children. Two key questions to ask are whether board meetings are held and if parents are welcome to attend. Some very effective programs welcome involvement by parents in a variety of ways and organize social events in which parents can interact with administrators and coaches.

**Costs and Commitments**

It's rare in this world to get something for nothing. Most programs require commitments of time and money. It's wise for parents to know the costs sooner rather than later. The costs can be financial—entry fees, equipment, uniforms, transportation for trips, contributions to fund-raisers, and so forth. In sports such as tennis, gymnastics, and figure skating, these costs can multiply rapidly in the form of private lessons and coaching, racket- or skating-club fees, and trips to distant meets. Many parents have found themselves in over their heads financially and unable to pull back because the child has become involved beyond the point of return. It's a good idea to ask parents who are already in the program for information.

Other costs may be in terms of time and emotional involvement. You can easily get into a program for your child's sake (or for your own hoped-for peace and quiet), only to find yourself stuck in a quicksand of time commitments. Suddenly, you're spending hours driving to practices and competitions, manning the hot dog booth, and going door-to-door selling candy bars. Those glorious days of working in the garden or watching the weekend ball games on TV are now a thing of the past.

Now, you may well make the choice to be time-involved, but to make an informed decision, you should try to find out:

- How many practices and competitions per week are there?
- Where are they held?
- Who provides transportation?
- Is there carpooling?
- What responsibilities are expected of parents? For example, are they expected to organize fund-raisers or to participate in field maintenance?
- Are allowances made for family vacations during the season, or will your family's vacation have to be postponed or canceled?
- Will your child have time for other activities? Obviously, if practices are held every night for two hours, there will be little time for other pursuits.
- Do practice and competition schedules interfere with dinnertime, homework, religious observances, or family outings?
- How long does the season last? In warm climates, youth baseball try-outs can begin as early as January, making for a far longer season than in snowbound regions.

### Program Philosophy and Objectives

The philosophy and values underlying a program can mean the difference between a positive experience and a negative one for your child. These values influence the goals that are set and the approaches used to pursue them. In Chapter 1, we stressed the crucial differences between the professional model and the developmental model of sports. It is important to keep these differences in mind as you examine a program.

> The professional sport model operates on the premise that winning is everything, whereas the developmental model insists that kids are everything.

Although we believe that the psychological and physical welfare of child athletes is best served in programs that emphasize participation, fun, and personal growth, we also recognize that some parents and children prefer win-oriented programs, even at very early ages. At the high school level, virtually all programs emphasize athletic excellence and winning. It is a parent's right to choose such a program, but it is also the parent's responsibility to make sure that winning is not emphasized at the sacrifice of the young athlete's interests. Many cases of athletic burnout result from pressures created by program philosophies that place winning first and athletes second.

The underlying philosophies of national youth sport organizations invariably emphasize athletes' personal growth and development through sports. However, at a local level, programs can vary in their commitment to the principles of the larger organization. Therefore, it is important to examine each program on an individual basis and to talk with parents whose children have been in the programs.

In examining a particular program, you may wish to get answers to the following questions:

- Does the program have a written statement of its goals and philosophy that is available to parents? If so, are they consistent with your needs?
- Is participation for everyone emphasized? Do all youngsters who turn out get a chance to play? Do some players get cut? Are there rules requiring that all children on a team get a certain amount of playing time?
- Is competition kept in perspective? Is competition seen as deadly serious business or as a contest in which to have fun? Are players taught to regard their opponents as enemies or as friendly challengers who make the contest possible?

- Are the needs of athletes taken into account in making decisions about such things as the time and length of practices and competitions? Are there attempts to match teams on the basis of size and ability for safe and equal competition?
- Are youngsters treated fairly? Do all children receive attention and instruction, or only the best performers? Is the emphasis on giving every child a good experience or on developing a select group of gifted athletes for higher levels of competition?
- Are attempts made to teach children sportsmanship and moral values? Is social and emotional development promoted?
- Are the rewards of participation viewed in terms of personal and team improvement or in the form of trophies, victory banquets, and all-star teams? Is the most improved athlete as important to the program as the most valuable athlete?

**Program Safety**

The physical well-being of your youngster is surely of concern in choosing a program. There will always be injuries in sports, but a safety-conscious program can help keep the risks at a minimum.

Highly desirable programs emphasize the importance of a medical examination prior to participating, and most programs require it. Children who have a physical condition that places them at high risk can often be identified and saved from injury. Several medical studies have shown preparticipation physical examinations to be associated with a lower rate of serious injuries.

Recognizing the value of screening examinations, some programs have contracted with sports medicine clinics or with individual physicians to make the exams less costly for parents. It is wise to inquire about this when selecting a program.

The safety of participants is increased when a program has developed safety rules for practices and competitions and when such rules are strictly enforced. Playing areas should be kept safe and free from hazards, such as holes, rocks, and broken glass. Your inquiry into these matters helps to draw necessary attention to them.

Try as we might to prevent them, injuries will occur and occasionally they will be serious ones. It is therefore important that coaches or adult supervisors who are trained in first aid be present at practices and competitions. There should also be established procedures to follow in case of an emergency.

> Safety-conscious programs have leaders who are prepared to deal quickly and effectively with injuries and emergencies when they occur.

Everyone is aware of the rising costs of health care and the resulting need to have insurance protection. Some programs require accident insurance for all participants. Several insurance groups offer athletic accident insurance to youth sport programs at reasonable rates. You should inquire about such coverage when considering a program. If the program does not subscribe to injury insurance, be certain that your own insurance provides adequate coverage for sport-related injuries to your youngster.

The likelihood of injuries increases when participants vary greatly in size, strength, and maturity. It is the smaller, less-developed athlete who is at greater risk under such circumstances. Research has shown that injuries can be reduced in collision sports, such as football or hockey, by matching participants in terms of size rather than by relying simply on age. Such matching not only reduces injuries but also gives all participants a greater opportunity to enjoy success and fair competition.

### The Quality of Leadership

Without doubt, the most important factor determining the outcome of your child's sport experience is the quality of adult supervision. The relationship that develops between your youngster and the coach or manager can become a very important one in your child's life. This adult will not only teach your child the techniques of the sport, but will also create a psychological climate that can have long-term effects. Coaches communicate important attitudes and values, and they serve as role models for children at an impressionable time in their lives.

Anytime you place your child in the hands of another adult, you should have confidence that he or she has what it takes to shoulder the responsibilities. Remember, most community-sponsored programs are staffed by volunteers who are sincerely interested in children. But this interest must be accompanied by knowledge of the sport and of children's needs.

> The most effective coaches are not only good teachers but good amateur psychologists as well.

Many youth sport administrators now recognize that they have a responsibility to prepare coaches for their leadership role. They also realize that instruction in the technical aspects of the sport is not enough. Workshops and clinics should focus on how to create a good psychological environment for personal and social growth and how to promote the physical safety of participants. The quality of a program is thus based in part on how well coaches are trained and evaluated. No matter what the program's potential may be, a subpar coach can ruin an otherwise good experience.

Before the season begins and while you're looking into a program, you may not know much about who will be coaching your youngster. At this point, about all you can do is to ask whether the coaches have preseason training or have gone through a certification program. Once the season begins, however, you will have opportunities to observe the coach. This is your right and your responsibility.

What should you look for in a coach? Here is a short checklist of qualities that are important in a youth sport coach:

*Knowledge and Teaching Skills*
- Does the coach know the rules and techniques of the sport? Can he communicate these to children?
- Does she demonstrate how to perform and give clear explanations?
- Are practices and competitions well organized, safe, and fun for the children?
- Is instruction matched to the age and knowledge level of the children?

*Motives and Philosophy*
- Does the coach seem to have a sincere interest in youngsters, or is coaching an ego trip?
- Does she put winning and losing in perspective? Is the focus where it should be—on fun, participation for all, and learning?
- Does the coach teach values as well as skills?
- Can he communicate his coaching philosophy to athletes and parents?

> Good leaders are like referees and umpires: they go
> practically unnoticed when doing their job right.

*Coaching Style*
- Does the coach try to motivate athletes through encouragement and praise, or do punishment and criticism dominate?
- Does the coach seem enthusiastic and enjoy relating to her athletes? Does she have fun?
- Are substitutes given as much attention as the stars, or are they ignored and made to feel inferior?
- Does the coach keep things well organized and prevent misbehavior, or does he let things get out of hand and have to scold the children to maintain control?

- Does the coach recognize and praise good effort even when things are not going well?
- Does the coach ask for input from athletes and listen to it, or does she call all the shots?
- Can the coach control his own emotions, or does he lose his cool with athletes or officials and provide a poor role model?

### Relationship Skills

- Is the coach sensitive to the individual needs and feelings of her athletes?
- Can he be flexible and know when everybody should *not* be treated exactly alike?
- Can she generate respect without demanding it and show respect for her athletes, officials, and opponents?
- Is he fair and consistent in his expectations of athletes?
- Can she communicate effectively with youngsters at their level?
- Do athletes he has coached wish to play for him again?
- Does she take the time and effort to communicate with parents, and is she open to their input?

Obviously no sport program is going to be perfect, since all are run by fallible human beings who make mistakes from time to time. You can't expect to get answers to every question presented above. But weighing the pros and cons can help you increase the chances of selecting the best program for your youngster and starting your young athlete on the road to a good sport experience.

# 5

# Nutrition and Young Athletes

## *Food for Sport*

Few things regularly raise more questions in the minds of parents of young athletes than concerns about how and what they should eat. As Mom wonders whether or not the children are really getting a balanced diet, Dad knows that if Carla and Brian would only eat better, they surely would play better. The professional nutritionist says that all the athlete needs is a generous balanced diet; the media tell about the professional tennis star who takes hundreds of food-supplement pills each day. To whom do you listen? How does one best satisfy the nutrition needs of active young competitors? Nothing less than optimal nutrition will be acceptable to the highly competitive athlete. They know that their diet does indeed have something important to do with performance in sports.

### UNIQUE NUTRITION NEEDS OF THE YOUNG ATHLETE

Active, energy-expending sport participation creates two and only two unique nutrition requirements: a need for increased food-energy intake to meet the needs of training and competition and an increased demand for water intake to replace the sweat lost during exercise. Satisfying these needs is essential for good performance as well as for the health and safety of the athlete. In addition, the young preadolescent and the older adolescent athlete have important growth needs that must be met.

Eating satisfies four vital needs. These are especially important for the growing youngster and take on additional importance for the physically active participant in sports:

- to provide energy
- to supply chemical building blocks for growth and repair of body tissues
- to supply essential chemicals needed for a host of body functions
- to satisfy important psychosocial needs through interaction with family and friends during mealtime

Living in a food-sufficient society, the majority of American young people have food available in abundance to satisfy the first three needs. Unfortunately, however, those who live in poverty do not have access to adequate diets—a problem of continuing importance and concern to all of us. The fourth need, to satisfy social and behavioral requirements that are met through the eating process, is of increasing concern. Loss of mealtime patterns, the changing family composition, and changing lifestyles all raise questions as to whether young people, even in a food-abundant environment, are getting an adequate diet and the security, education, and learning experiences that come from mealtime contact with family and friends.

> The quality of the diet is directly proportionate to the quality of the environment in which it is eaten.

For most Americans, eating in a pleasant place with amiable people essentially guarantees that the nutritional quality of their diet will be very high and more than adequate. (One would like to always believe that the most pleasant place and most amiable people would be at the family table.) Eating alone or on the run is the surest way to eat badly. Unfortunately, too many young athletes and families eat this way.

## THE YOUNG ATHLETE'S DIET

Parents are keenly aware that the elementary school–aged child has to "eat right to grow right," but a new dimension of food need has been introduced into the parenting concerns of many families: how to feed a growing boy or girl who is now an athlete. In previous chapters, the goals of sport participation have been clearly spelled out—having fun, getting exercise, learning skills, making friends, and so forth. These goals are in no way in conflict with the goals of good nutrition for young athletes.

Actually, attempting to exploit sport interests of boys and girls for the purpose of getting them to eat more or differently can jeopardize the most important goal of youth sport participation—to have fun. The 10-year-old athlete should not be cajoled into eating three health-promoting meals a day simply to make him or her a better quarterback, second baseman, or figure skater. He or she should have an opportunity to eat those three meals to make him or her a healthy 10-year-old. Sport interests should not be used as a weapon at mealtime. It is the parents' responsibility to ensure that a proper perspective is maintained.

Concerned parents determine *what* the young athlete will eat. Nature will direct the young athlete as to *how much* to eat.

Youth sport participation by the preadolescent should not be such an intense experience that satisfying excessive energy expenditures is an unduly great concern. However, monitoring water needs during practices and competitions is becoming an increasing problem as young athletes become more active in intensely competitive situations where temperature and humidity are high. The specific needs and hazards of fluid replacement in athletes will be considered later in this chapter. It is a common problem in the more intense activities of older athletes, but there is a very real need to be alert to the fluid requirements of the elementary school–aged athlete as well.

## HOW SPORTS CAN INTERFERE WITH GOOD NUTRITION

Can youth sport participation interfere with the good nutrition and good growth that result from healthy eating during childhood? "With a girl in gymnastics and two boys in soccer and baseball," said one parent, "mealtime eating together is a matter of historical interest in our family."

We sincerely believe that a good sport experience is important for growing up healthy in today's society. But we recognize that there are other needs, priorities, and growth-promoting requirements of a happy, healthy childhood. Yes, there is life beyond sports! Before family life and mealtime disappear from your household, we suggest that you hold a family council with your children, define the goals of youth sports, and then preserve a generous number of those valuable weekends, mealtimes, and other times for being together as a family.

It is equally important to be alert to the impact of more intense, competitive sport participation on the dietary needs of the adolescent athlete during his or her high school years.

Scott was sent to a sports medicine clinic because of a rather rapid deterioration in performance with his high school swim team. It was early in the preseason, and already Scott seemed to be "stale." He had no specific complaints that suggested he might be ill, but he did state that he had lost between 11 and 13 pounds during the first 2 months of training. His grades in school were great—straight As—but he was getting very worried about his swim performance.

Scott was a good swimmer—state high school champion last year and ranked nationally this year. He had decided to take this year to find out just how good he could be. He was swimming up to 20,000 meters a day (about 12 miles), doing his academic work, and volunteering two evenings a week as a clerk in a storefront health clinic. He "usually" ate lunch, seldom ate breakfast, and "got dinner somewhere" every evening. Although a very intelligent young man, Scott couldn't (or wouldn't) understand why he was losing weight and underperforming. The fact was that his food-energy intake was simply inadequate to meet the very generous energy expenditures of his active lifestyle and extremely demanding training schedule.

Food-energy intake insufficient to satisfy the demands of growth, training, and daily school activities is the most common nutrition-related problem encountered among young athletes. Like Scott, some athletes become overcommitted to an extent that their lifestyles allow no time for eating. Others come from disorganized families in which food is not regularly available or from impoverished homes in which there is no adequate food supply. Whatever the reason might be, when energy intake is inadequate to meet the needs of the active young male or female athlete, there will be involuntary weight loss. And it is inevitable that the athlete will experience deterioration in performance. Recorded weighing once or twice each week will identify the athlete whose diet is inadequate to meet energy needs.

> Maintaining a stable desired weight assures that food energy intakes are sufficient to satisfy energy demands.

Three groups of athletes most likely to experience involuntary weight loss and poor training performance are swimmers, wrestlers, and basketball players. These high-energy-expending individuals may find that three meals a day plus a generous evening snack are not enough to satisfy their energy needs. If a larger diet does not stabilize competing weight during the season and if adding extra meals or snacks is unacceptable to the athlete in question, the use of a convenient liquid food can be helpful by providing 500 to 1,000 kilocalories of additional food energy each day. High-energy drinks are included in these products. This is one of the very few legitimate uses of a good supplement in sports. Taking in sufficient total food energy is essential in meeting the optimal nutrition needs of even the most sophisticated athlete.

In meeting the energy needs of the active young athlete, one should pay attention to the appropriate distribution of energy intake

throughout the day. It is not uncommon to encounter athletes underperforming in afternoon practice sessions after having eaten no
breakfast and only catch-as-catch-can lunch from the corridor vending machine. The lack of ability of these athletes to perform between
3:00 and 5:00 in the afternoon should come as no surprise. The body
has very limited ability to store its most readily available energy in the
form of carbohydrates before it is converted to body fat. Body fat is
a less efficient source of energy, as it must be mobilized from fat de-
posits and transferred to muscle cells before it can serve as an energy
source for muscle work. Individuals who perform vigorous physical
work during the day have always found regular food-energy intake
spaced at intervals to be essential to good performance.

## EATING THE RIGHT FOODS

A varied diet sufficient in amount to satisfy energy needs will provide
all of the essential nutrients the young athlete needs. Young athletes,
their coaches, and particularly their parents are continually questioning
the adequacy of the athlete's diet in providing all of those nutrients that
are known to be essential for good health and athletic performance.
Actually, there are approximately 60 substances recognized as so-called
essential nutrients—substances that must be included in the daily diet.
New dietary customs, fast foods, meatless diets, and skipped meals all
raise questions as to whether the young woman or young man active
in sports is adequately satisfying nutritional needs. Many coaches are
asking, "Can you really 'do your thing' with a hamburger, fries, and a
shake on Friday night, a pizza on Saturday, and another fast-food dinner another night during the week?" In one nutrition study, 35 percent
of a population of high school varsity basketball players ate their evening meal alone the night before they were interviewed. As we've noted
before, eating alone is likely to mean that you will not eat well.

Another factor that causes parents and coaches concern is the con-
troversy surrounding special diets and dietary supplements. Some self-
declared nutrition "experts" claim that without a particular miracle diet

and/or supplement, we all run the risk of being chronically undernourished. Others promote the healing or empowering properties of certain herbs, remedies, or vitamins. It is difficult for the average adult—let alone a young athlete—to even sort out those claims. The "bottom line" here is that such nutritional solutions are not only useless and expensive but perhaps dangerous. It is best to consult a physician or a legitimate nutritional specialist if there is real concern about nutrition needs.

> Applying a simple diet evaluation scheme is the athlete's best protection against getting involved with useless, expensive, and dangerous supplements.

How the athlete ensures the adequacy of his or her diet is important and can be the best protection against needless and expensive nutrient supplements. A straightforward and effective system of diet evaluation can be used by any parent or young athlete. Merely write down all of the food items eaten each day for three or four typical days. Then see if there are included in that diet appropriate representations of the four food groups that, most of us have learned, are essential to good diets:

- Each day, are there *two* servings of *dairy foods* (e.g., milk, cheese, ice cream, yogurt)?
- Are there *two* servings of *high-protein foods* (e.g., meats, fish, poultry, legumes, beans)?
- Are there *four* servings of *fruits or vegetables*?
- Are there *four* servings of cereal and *grain foods* (e.g., bread, baked goods)?

When these 12 servings are included in each day's diet, the athlete and parent can be confident that the intake of all the known essential nutrients is adequate to meet the needs of even the athlete who is training heavily. This diet makes any vitamin, mineral, protein, or other food supplement unnecessary.

A sports medicine physician told us two high school athletes were seen in his office on successive days with very similar complaints. Both were feeling unwell, with marked bone pain and severe pounding headaches that kept them awake at night and prevented them from attending classes. This unusual combination of symptoms alerted the physician to ask whether the students had been taking any vitamin pills or supplements. Indeed they had been. Both were candidates for the football team in the upcoming autumn and were trying to "bulk up" to increase their weight and potential for making the team. They were each taking three cans daily of a liquid vitamin-and-protein mixture. Laboratory tests demonstrated that they were both suffering from vitamin A poisoning, a serious, painful intoxication that takes many weeks to get over. In Chapter 9, we will outline safe and effective ways to increase playing weight for improved performance in certain sports. These do not include taking expensive and potentially dangerous protein-and-vitamin supplements unless prescribed by a physician.

> Vitamin, protein, mineral, and amino acid supplements are useless and needlessly expensive for the healthy young athlete.

Once again, the athlete's diet that contains twelve servings with appropriate representation from the four food groups makes supplements unnecessary. But it will not meet the energy needs of *all* athletes. For some youngsters, this basic four-food-group diet must be supplemented with second servings and preference foods to meet what may be very generous energy requirements:

- A good rule to follow is to eat first what you need (the 12 servings from the four food groups), then eat what you want to satisfy energy demands.
- A second rule is that if and when your diet is so inadequate that you need a vitamin or protein supplement, then you don't need a supplement, you need a better diet. The athlete can never compete on a diet of pills and powders.

## MEETING THE ATHLETE'S NEED FOR WATER AND SALT

In addition to the athlete's unique need for increased intake of food energy to meet the demands of training and competing, another specific need of the athlete is replacement of the water lost in sweating. A large young athlete can lose ten or more pounds of water during an intense practice session. Basketball players in an air-conditioned gym lose four to six pounds of body water during a typical high school practice. Replacing these losses is critical both to continued good performance and avoidance of serious heat disorders, such as cramps, heat exhaustion, and heat stroke.

Body water is involved in several functions critical to performance. The body's chemical processes that provide the energy for muscle work occur in water. All of the transport functions of oxygen, nutrients, and body wastes are carried on in body water. Of most importance to the exercising athlete is the fact that the large amount of heat generated by exercising muscles is transported by water in the blood to the skin, where water is essential for the production of sweat. Body heat is dissipated most efficiently through the evaporation of sweat on exposed skin surfaces. An abundant supply of body water, first to transport muscle-generated heat and then to produce the sweat needed for evaporative cooling, is the best insurance against the complications of heat cramps, heat exhaustion, and life-threatening heat stroke.

Losses of body water of as little as 2 percent of total body weight (3 pounds for a 150-pound athlete, for example) will cause a very noticeable decrease in performance. With such water loss, energy production is compromised and endurance is limited. Preventing excessive body-water deficits by fluid intake prior to exercise and at intervals during exercise will contribute measurably to performance.

Early one September Monday morning, the telephone in a sports medicine clinic rang. On the line were a father, a mother, and a 16-year-old daughter, each on his or her own telephone extension. The daughter was a nationally ranked junior tennis champion who had just been defeated in the Midwest tennis championships played in St. Louis the preceding weekend. She had repeatedly defeated the person she lost the championship to, but on this particular Sunday she faded badly as the match progressed.

This had been a most disappointing performance. In the opinion of her father, the tennis player had not eaten right, and he had decided that she should be "talked to" about her diet. Mother wondered if she should be taking more vitamins. Neither concern would appear to have caused her to blow a particular tennis match. You don't get to the Midwest championship finals if you are suffering from malnutrition.

During the conversation, the physician asked the daughter to weigh herself. She came back to report that some 16 hours after her disastrous match, she weighed 8 or 9 pounds less than her normal pretournament weight. Playing in the heat of a St. Louis September weekend, she had not monitored her needs for water, had lost more than 10 pounds of body water, became dehydrated, and underperformed. She admitted to a rather severe, throbbing headache and feeling faint for several hours after the match, an early symptom of impending heat exhaustion.

Exercise scientists have studied the nature of sweat and have discovered some very interesting and important findings for the athlete. Sweat is a very dilute body fluid when compared to other body fluids. It contains less than one-third the concentration of salts that blood plasma contains, for example. It is interesting that the better conditioned the athlete, the more dilute and watery the sweat. When athletes sweat, they lose much more water than salt.

> Sweating results in an increase in the concentration
> of the body's salts and minerals.

Other interesting things that have been learned about sweat is that women have fewer sweat glands and produce less sweat than men. They have greater skin surface area for every pound of body weight, however, and unlike men, they dissipate more of the heat generated in exercise by convection and conduction from the skin than by evaporation. In contrast to what was thought many years ago, women tolerate exercise in hot environments as well as men.

Prior to the onset of adolescence, children do not produce sweat efficiently. They have a limited capacity for evaporative heat loss from their bodies during exercise. However, it has been shown that they make a very early psychological adjustment to exertion in the heat, not noticing it as much as older individuals, even though their bodies' mechanisms for dissipating heat are poorly developed. This puts the young athlete at increased risk to heat exhaustion. Preventing heat disorders in very young athletes is an increasing concern, as large numbers of preadolescent sport participants find themselves exercising in competitive situations in the heat of summer and early autumn. These youngsters must have their practices and competitions modified or rescheduled during hot weather and have their fluid needs and the intensity of play carefully monitored. Indeed, these athletes will be the last to know when they are at risk to heat exhaustion or even heat stroke.

> The increased risk of heat exhaustion of very young athletes demands the attention of parents and coaches.

*Water is the ideal beverage for replacing the fluid losses of the sweating athlete.* The water should be refrigerator temperature, plentiful, and provided in a sanitary container. So-called sport drinks present several problems for the athlete losing body water through sweat. Sport drinks contain a variety of salts that when added to the body only increase the already elevated salt concentration of the dehydrated athlete. The concentration of salts and the masking sugar flavor cause these beverages to leave the stomach slowly, producing a sense of fullness and satiety. This actually discourages the athlete from taking in much-needed water. In addition, in the intense emotional environment of competition, all senses become more sensitive, making the distinctive flavor of certain beverages unpleasant and discouraging the intake of water.

With no such disadvantages, water remains a wonderfully inexpensive, ideal beverage for replacing the water losses of sweat. Every sailor knows that you don't maintain hydration by drinking saltwater, but American merchandisers have sold salty water in plastic bottles to millions of athletes.

Athletes can very effectively monitor their needs for water replacement by recognizing that any weight that is lost in a period of a few hours or even a few days is essentially all water weight. With a pound of fat the equivalent of 3,500 kilocalories of energy, and the energy expenditure to run one mile approximately 100 calories, it is apparent that any sudden changes in weight are not due to a significant change in the body's fat content. Nude weighing before and after each game or match and drinking sufficient water to maintain a stable precompetition weight are highly desirable procedures. During daily or two-a-day practices of any sport in warm, humid weather, it is recommended that all athletes record a nude weight before and after each practice. This is the surest way to be certain that fluid losses are replaced between practice sessions.

Tasting the salt in the perspiration running off the fevered brow during exercise obviously generates some real concern on the part of the athlete as to how these salt losses are to be replaced. Thus, many athletes are impressed with the much-promoted salt- and electrolyte-containing sport drinks. Fortunately, there has been some very elaborate research on this at outstanding exercise-physiology laboratories. These investigations document that *all of the salt and mineral losses of the most profusely sweating athlete are abundantly replaced by the elements in the generous mixed diet of the exercising athlete.* The kidneys sort out what of this dietary intake is needed for replacement of sweat losses and what can be excreted as waste into the urine. Taking extra minerals in drinks or salt tablets only taxes the body's normal mechanisms for maintaining a healthy mineral balance. Particularly threatening is the use of salt tablets, which athletes might take indiscriminately. Some time ago, a football heat-stroke victim was found to have fourteen salt tablets in his stomach on X-ray examination—salt that only accentuated the consequences of his severe dehydration.

Clean, cool water is the ideal beverage for athletes.

Young athletes should drink lots of clean, cool water. Drinking 8 to 10 ounces immediately before playing delays the harmful effects of sweat loss. Additionally, coaches should be reminded to schedule frequent water breaks, and athletes should be encouraged to ask for water. In hot weather, water breaks should be scheduled every 25 minutes, and generous amounts of water should be readily available to young athletes.

## EATING BEFORE AND DURING COMPETITION

The psychological effect of the pregame meal should not be minimized or ignored. It can serve the needs of the athlete and the team to exploit the very real emotional impact of food and eating together. An important thing about planning the pregame meal should be kept in mind: it should be planned! A well-planned eating experience tells athletes that they are being well prepared to handle their responsibilities in the upcoming competition. Here are guidelines for planning the pregame meal for an athlete or a team:

- Locate a suitable place where the team or athletes can be together and can concentrate on the upcoming competition.
- The meal is best if it is low in fat, modest in protein, and high in carbohydrate (bread, spaghetti, macaroni, potatoes, pancakes, cereals, fruits, vegetables).
- The meal should be modest in amount.
- The menu should avoid those foods that carry a greater-than-usual risk of food poisoning, such as cream gravies, turkey, and cream pastries.
- Fatty foods are slower and more difficult to digest. Thus, they should be eaten five or more hours before a competitive event.

Having had nothing to eat for several hours, many athletes will play "hungry." An old rule applies here: *Saturday's game is played on*

*Wednesday, Thursday, and Friday's food intake.* The pregame meal is not the time to try to provide all of the energy for some high-energy-expending competition.

| |
|---|
| **A big steak dinner is a poor choice as a pregame meal.** |

A very simple pregame menu that is not expensive and can be eaten 2.5 to 3 hours before the competition includes the following:

- lean beef or chicken sandwiches
- fruit punch or fruit juice
- a large Jell-O salad
- nutrition bars or generous servings of sherbet

As young athletes become increasingly serious about their sport commitments, there are those who direct their precompetition anxieties to their stomachs and upper gastrointestinal tracts. They may experience precompetition diarrhea or be pregame vomiters. These delightfully intense individuals can profit by being introduced to complete liquid pregame meals. These products typically come in small cans, which can be chilled and sipped up to 1 or 2 hours before competition time. Certain athletes find these products the answer to food intake during daylong competition, such as track meets, gymnastics competitions, and wrestling tournaments.

In addition to the above, special attention should be given to the food needs of young athletes when they are away from home and spending an evening in a motel. "On the road" athletes are at considerable risk for gastronomical disasters and compromised performance the following day. It is as important to plan evening eating as it is to plan pregame food intake. Nutrition bars and sherbet make good high-carbohydrate evening snacks. By providing such refreshments, athletes can be kept away from vending machines and fast-food establishments and make a positive contribution to the energy taken into the next day's competition.

# Sport Injuries

## *When the Colors of Sports Are Black and Blue*

Serious injuries are not common in sports. This is particularly true for athletes less than 14 years of age. Their small size and limited strength and assertiveness combine with safety rules and adult supervision to help minimize the risk of significant injury. Sport injuries become more common in high school, where the intensity of competition increases along with the size and strength of the participants.

> Older and stronger athletes are more capable of causing injury to themselves and to their opponents.

Fortunately, regardless of age, most athletes will not suffer serious sport injuries, and when properly managed, injuries will limit training and competition for no more than a few days. Because responsibility for the recognition and management of sport-related injuries often falls on parents, there is some essential information that you should have about their nature and treatment.

### WHAT IS A SPORT INJURY?

The sore muscles Dad suffered the morning after a 3-hour volleyball game at last summer's office picnic is not technically a sport injury.

Those hurts are merely Nature's way of telling Dad that he should probably do some regular physical exercise. There are certain symptoms, however, that indicate a true sport injury and should be recognized as such by athletes, coaches, and parents. These include:

- bleeding
- mental confusion or loss of consciousness
- numbness or tingling of an extremity
- a recognizable deformity of any body part
- instability of any joint, such as a knee that "wobbles"
- the sound of tearing or ripping at the time of injury
- localized swelling or pain
- absence of a full range of motion of any joint

An athlete with any of these symptoms should not return to play or practice until a very specific diagnosis of the nature of the injury has been made and the symptoms of injury have completely disappeared. Any of these injuries can easily be made worse by continued participation. Unable to move normally and protect themselves when injured, athletes with any of these symptoms are at high risk to a new injury.

> The most common sport-related injuries are the so-called overuse injuries, the too-much, too-soon, too-fast injuries.

Overuse injuries result from the improper or excessive use of some body part, most often tendons and muscles. Overuse injuries are often identified with certain sports or types of activities. There is the jogger's heel, the jumper's knee, the tennis elbow, the swimmer's shoulder, the Little League elbow, and so on. All are the result of overuse of a specified muscle or tendon unit in training for a certain sport.

In collision sports, such as football, wrestling, ice hockey, and lacrosse, the most common injuries are bumps, bruises, and lacerations. In both collision and running sports, muscles, tendons, and ligaments can be stretched or torn in strains and sprains, although most of these possible injuries tend to be minor ones.

The injured athlete or the parents of the youth sport participant must assume some responsibility for the proper management of a sport injury, initiating and following a safe and effective management plan that will assure the athlete's return to participation as quickly and as safely as possible. Prompt treatment and effective follow-through on a sound treatment plan are most important. Postponing care or failing to follow the prescribed treatment plan will prolong discomfort, hamper performance, and greatly increase the risk of reinjury.

Athletes should be instructed to inform their coach or the athletic trainer about any injury immediately, so that they can be promptly treated and returned to the practice or competition as soon as possible. Attempting to "tough it out" and play through pain can harm both the athlete and the team. It is better to stay out of practice for 2 or 3 days while an injury is being properly treated and return to action only when fully recovered.

### THINGS *NOT* TO DO AFTER A SPORT INJURY
Here are some important don'ts to emphasize to your young athlete:

- *Don't* try to hide an injury. Report the injury to the coach or trainer.
- *Don't* apply treatment other than simple first aid until a specific diagnosis has been made by the trainer or a doctor.
- *Don't* apply heat to an injury without orders from the doctor. A common but mistaken belief is that heat helps a new injury. By increasing swelling, it can actually make things worse rather than better.
- *Don't* use an injured part if it hurts. More pain means more injury.
- *Don't* take any drugs unless they are prescribed by a physician.
- *Don't* tape or splint an injured part without specific instructions from a doctor.
- *Don't* go back to practice or competition until you have a full range of motion, full strength (both sides are equally strong), and full function of the injured part.

These don'ts should be modified only under the direct orders of a physician or a certified trainer (not a volunteer or student trainer). The quickest and safest way to get back into active participation is to limit activity as long as there is any pain or swelling, then to follow rigidly the prescribed rehabilitation program, which will include a schedule of specifically planned exercises. In specialized sport medicine clinics, the patient problem most frequently seen is the athlete with an inadequately rehabilitated sport injury who returned to his or her sport and was re-injured. In a large study of high school football injuries, 50 percent of those injured were reinjured when they returned to participation—a sad commentary on injury management.

## THINGS TO DO AFTER A SPORT INJURY
The athlete's first responsibility when injured is to get out of the practice or competition. Continued participation may make the injury worse and may place the athlete at increased risk to another injury. A healthy substitute is better for the team than an injured all-star.

When leaving the field or court, the athlete should avoid using the injured part. This usually involves getting physical support from others so he or she won't walk on an injured leg or ankle. Additionally, an injured arm or wrist should be supported (with a sling if possible).

> Never apply heat to a sports injury unless
> it is ordered by a physician.

Promptly apply the only first-aid treatment that is safe for treatment of a sports injury without professional advice—*ICE* (*I* for ice, *C* for compression, and *E* for elevation). The *ICE* treatment is easily applied and easily available on the sidelines at practices and competitions. All that is needed are plastic bags (from the supermarket produce counter), crushed ice, and a picnic cooler, which holds the bags of crushed ice and some wet four-inch elastic bandages.

To apply the *ICE* treatment, remove any part of the uniform that surrounds the injured area and elevate the arm or leg above the level of the heart. Apply one layer of the cold, wet elastic bandage on the skin directly over the injury, put the plastic bag of ice on the bandage, and firmly wrap the remainder of the bandage around the bag of ice. Keep the ice and the compression wrap on the elevated, immobilized injury for 25 to 30 minutes. As long as there is pain and/or swelling, keep the injury elevated. Avoid standing or walking on a painful leg or ankle before or after the ice application. *ICE* treatment for 25 to 30 minutes may be applied four or more times a day for a few days following an injury. If pain or swelling persists, see a physician.

When a girl sprains her ankle in a basketball game and its supporting ligaments are stretched and torn, or when a wide receiver strains and ruptures the fibers of a hamstring muscle, a sequence of events occurs that is common to all such sport injuries. Blood vessels are damaged and some will break, allowing blood and fluid to accumulate in the injured area. This causes increased pressure, swelling, and pain, and the pressure and swelling cause further damage and injury to the surrounding tissues.

This reaction of the body to injury has a protective function as well. The pain of the initial injury causes the muscles of the injured area to go into further painful spasms. This limits movement and discourages the use of the injured area, thereby preventing further injury.

> When properly applied, *ICE* treatments
> can do no harm to any type of injury.

The *ICE* treatment helps in three important ways:

- First, applying ice chills the bruised or injured area, causing blood vessels to contract and reducing circulation to the injured area—quite the opposite of what heat applications might do.
- Second, applying pressure with the elastic bandage inhibits the accumulation of blood and fluids in the area, thereby minimizing painful and damaging swelling.

- Finally, elevating the injury decreases fluid accumulation in the injured area, puts the area at rest, and helps reduce painful muscle spasms.

When applied promptly and repeatedly, *ICE* treatments significantly reduce the discomfort and period of limited activity resulting from an injury. Almost anything else—including heat applications—can cause harm in some instances.

The story of Alex, a guard on a basketball team for 13- and 14-year-olds, is a case in point. He was playing in a city-wide postseason tournament when, in the middle of the second half, he broke free for a layup. As he came down from jumping, he tripped on the foot of a trailing opponent. He fell heavily, with his weight on the outer edge of his foot. It collapsed under him, painfully stretching and tearing portions of the ligaments on the outside of his left ankle.

The physician in attendance at the tournament examined the ankle, diagnosed a moderately severe sprain, and determined that an X-ray examination wasn't needed at the time. A volunteer trainer properly equipped with plastic ice bags and chilled, wet elastic bandages applied ice and compression to the injured ankle and had Alex elevate the ankle on an upper bleacher during the remainder of the game.

At the end of the game, supported by his teammates, Alex showered and was driven home, where 30-minute *ICE* treatments were applied three more times before bedtime. A suitcase was used to elevate the foot of Alex's bed while he slept. (A pillow under the ankle is not recommended; it only stays in place for about the first 3 minutes of sleep.)

Alex remained at home watching the NCAA basketball championships with his father during the weekend. He used crutches rented from a local pharmacy for essential movements and applied the *ICE* treatment every 3 hours for 30 minutes. On Monday he used the crutches to go to school, applied the *ICE* treatment in the nurse's office during his two free periods, and checked in with his physician after school. By now there remained only slight swelling and some discoloration around the injured ankle. When Alex could walk without pain, he was allowed limited "essential walking" without crutches and began a series of progressive muscle-strengthening exercises.

The spring soccer season was to start in 3 weeks, and thus Alex was conscientious about his rehabilitation program. By doing the ankle-strengthening exercises three times each day, he was able to begin jogging in a week, to do full running in 2 weeks, and to cut and do sharp turns in 3 weeks. Alex was able to work out with his soccer team in time. He had also learned how to wrap his ankle and was advised to do so when exercising for the next year.

Although it took nearly a month, this was an excellent recovery from a moderately severe ankle sprain—a very common injury. The rapid and complete recovery was the result of repeated use of the *ICE* treatment, support and crutches to avoid further injury to the area, and the program of rehabilitation exercises. Alex's future participation in sport will not be limited by a persistent weak ankle of which so many athletes complain.

Should an athlete be allowed to play when injured or ill? Absolutely not! The only time that it is justified to play an injured or ill youngster is when winning is more important than the child's health—which, of course, should *never* be the case!

> Never encourage an athlete to play with pain, for there is a strong possibility of making the injury more serious.

How do you know when an injury or illness is sufficiently severe to remove a youngster from competition or to withhold your child from a practice or competition? The decision should be based on a strong dose of common sense. And if you are uncertain about it, be sure to consult with a physician.

## WHEN INJURY PREVENTS PARTICIPATION

A young athlete may be temporarily or permanently eliminated from a sport program because of an injury. This can be frustrating. For example, a youngster with promising athletic ability can have future hopes dashed by a severe knee or back injury. In such instances, parents must (a) try to understand the feelings of frustration, (b) put up with occasional expressions of this frustration, and (c) support the youngster through a difficult period. Recognize also that depression, even if not openly expressed, may be reflected in loss of appetite, disturbed sleep patterns, or general apathy. If such symptoms continue or become severe, professional counseling should be pursued.

> **Sport injuries can take an emotional**
> **as well as physical toll on athletes.**

If a severe injury occurs to your young athlete, it is very important that he or she be seen by a sports medicine specialist. Most larger communities have specialized sports medicine clinics devoted to diagnosis, treatment, and rehabilitation. What else might be done?

- A coach can make sure the injured athlete is included in team practices and competitions in some way. For example, an injured softball player can coach the bases or keep the scorebook.
- Injured athletes who cannot participate actively during practice can use imagery to mentally practice their skills. Many injured athletes have reported that they maintained their skill level or even performed at a higher level when they returned because of the use of mental rehearsal.

## PREVENTING SPORT INJURIES
Everyone involved in youth sports—coaches, athletes, administrators, and parents—should constantly seek practical ways to minimize the risk of sport injury. Here are some things you can do to reduce the risk of injury:

- Assure that competition is between persons with similar levels of proficiency, maturity, size, and strength. This is particularly important in the collision sports, where the risk of injury is greatest. The less-skilled and smaller players get more than their share of injuries in such sports.

- Be sure that athletes are at appropriate levels of conditioning before they turn out for practice or attempt vigorous competition. A good idea for athletes is to talk to the coach 2 or 3 months prior to the first workouts and get suggestions for a preseason conditioning program. The unconditioned athlete gets injured early in the season, sometimes seriously.

- Be certain that protective equipment is available and used. Protective equipment has been developed and provided for good reasons. Be sure that it fits, that it doesn't need repair, and that it is used properly.

- Most sports are played on the feet. Be certain that shoes and socks fit and that socks are clean and without holes. Many troublesome foot problems can be prevented.

- Don't allow athletes to wear jewelry in active sports. Neck jewelry can be dangerous; rings can produce serious finger injury by getting caught in basket nets, uniforms, and so on.

- Make sure athletes practice good hygiene. Skin infections are common among athletes and can keep them out of training for a week or more of expensive treatment. They can also spread to other team members. Showering with an antibacterial soap daily is a good practice to reduce the risk of skin infections. Keep all uniforms laundered and clean.

- Fingernails should always be trimmed shorter than the tip of the finger to prevent painful scratches and potentially serious eye injuries. This is especially important in basketball.

- Never allow an athlete to play with a fever. Otherwise mild, common viral infections can become serious illnesses following a hard workout or competition. Stay home; the risk of passing an infection on to other team members should always be avoided. A good rule is that with fever over 100 degrees, stay home and get well.

- Whether at a school or community venue, take a minute to be sure that anything an athlete may run into or get injured from is well away from the playing area. Bicycles, automobiles, benches, lawn mowers, sprinklers, scorers' tables, and other obstacles can all cause serious injuries.

## BE PREPARED FOR AN EMERGENCY

Most injuries occurring in sports are minor, but on very rare occasions, serious, life-threatening injuries occur. These emergencies usually have to be managed on the scene before any medical help is available. In professionally supervised school sports, the coach or trainer will be responsible for a plan of action to be followed in an emergency. In community sport programs in which most children participate, there will be no professionally trained coach or trainer on hand.

In these situations we strongly recommend to volunteer coaches, parents, and athletes over the age of 12 that they do one thing before getting involved any further in sports: Get certified in CPR (cardiopulmonary resuscitation). CPR training is available through the American Red Cross, local fire departments, schools, or Boy/Girl Scout programs.

> Training in CPR teaches the basic life-saving techniques that can keep a seriously injured athlete alive until emergency medical help arrives.

An accident or injury to an athlete that results in any of the following symptoms presents a serious emergency that demands the skills of CPR training and prompt medical assistance:

- not breathing
- unconscious
- bleeding
- in shock—particularly during hot weather

Injured athletes in these conditions can die before medical assistance arrives on the scene if someone isn't prepared to initiate thoughtful action.

Before you as a parent attend your daughter or son's next practice or competition, take ten seconds and think through exactly how you would get emergency help if one of those very rare but life-threatening injuries should occur. You must know:

- Where is there a cellular phone or a landline?
- Whom do you call for help? (Dial 911.)
- What is the location of the field or gym?
- Will the emergency vehicle be able to get on the field? If there is a locked gate, who has the key?

If you don't know these things, you may be helpless when the crisis occurs. Someone's son or daughter or teammate could die because no one was prepared for the unexpected.

Earlier we listed some important don'ts for sport injuries in general. The following recommendations are even more critical because of the life-threatening nature of some serious injuries:

- *Don't* move an unconscious player any more than needed for CPR.
- *Don't* move any athlete who can't move all four extremities freely.
- *Don't* remove the helmet from any unconscious player. You may seriously compound a possible injury to the spine.
- *Don't* use ammonia capsules to attempt to revive an athlete who may be unconscious or "dinged." They can complicate a neck or spine injury and may cause face and eye burns.

Steve and his friends were to be the stalwarts of this year's local Babe Ruth baseball team. They decided to get together for an informal Saturday afternoon game the week before practice was to begin. Shortly after the game started, Steve raced for second base and slid headfirst toward the bag. As he slid, his left arm caught on the base and his legs became tangled with the feet of the second baseman, who was covering the bag. Steve's back bent in a severe arch. He heard a crack and felt an excruciating pain. As his teammates gathered around, he cried out that he couldn't move his legs. Brad, the catcher's father, took charge and ordered that no one move or even touch Steve. Brad dialed 911 on his cell phone and reported the following: "There has been an injury at the baseball diamond in Seahurst Park at Fifteenth and Collins streets. A player has hurt his back and can't move his legs."

In less than 5 minutes, medics were on the field. Steve was moved by expert medical-aid personnel and within minutes was in the hospital and being taken care of by specialists. Steve had broken a bone in his back, but his legs were not permanently paralyzed. He actually played the last four games of the season.

Lots of people say that Steve was very lucky. But Brad, Steve, Steve's parents, and his doctors know that luck had little to do with it. Someone—Brad—knew what to do and was prepared to do it. Steve was lucky all right—lucky that Brad was there, for the specialist told Steve's parents that he could easily have been paralyzed if he had been moved incorrectly.

Much of the fun and satisfaction of sport participation comes from extending oneself to maximum effort. Such stresses may on occasion result in injury. Although most injuries are not serious, they do interfere temporarily with one's ability to compete and can result in more serious injuries if not cared for properly. Know how to manage the more common, less severe injuries that will be brought home by young athletes. Don't let them become more severe than need be or lead to a needlessly prolonged period of disability.

# Athletic Stress

## Developing Coping Skills through Sports

Sport participation places both physical and psychological demands on athletes. From youth leagues to the professional level, athletes are forced to cope with the stresses that arise from competing head-on with others in activities that are important to the athletes and others, such as parents, coaches, and peers. Some athletes learn to cope successfully with these stresses, and for them sports are enjoyable and challenging. Others who are unable to cope find sport participation to be a stressful and threatening experience.

There is no question that people differ in their ability to cope successfully with stressful situations. Such differences result primarily from the attitudes and coping skills that are learned during the childhood and adolescent years. Athletics can be an important arena in which such skills are learned. In a sense, the athletic experience can be a sort of laboratory for trying out and mastering ways of dealing with stress.

Through their athletic experiences, youngsters can develop attitudes, beliefs, and coping skills that carry over into other areas of their lives. Childhood is the best time to learn stress-management skills, and in this chapter we are concerned with what you as a parent can do to help in this process.

## WHAT IS STRESS?

Before discussing ways of reducing stress, we need to explore what we mean by stress. An examination of what stress is should give us some clues on how to cope successfully with it.

We typically use the term *stress* in two different but related ways. First, we use the term to refer to *situations* in our lives that place physical or psychological demands on us. Family conflicts, work pressures, or school problems are examples of events that might cause us to say, "There is a lot of stress in my life right now."

The second way in which we use the term is to refer to our mental, emotional, and behavioral *responses* to these demanding situations. Worry, anger, tension, and depression are examples of such reactions, as are loss of appetite, sleep difficulties, and inability to get one's mind off the problem. We are referring to such reactions when we say, "I'm feeling a lot of stress right now."

In figure 7.1, we present an analysis of stress that takes both the situation and the person's reactions into account. As you can see, four major elements are involved.

The first element is the external situation that is making some sort of physical or psychological demand on the person. Typically we view our emotions as being directly triggered by these "pressure" situations, as shown in such statements as "He makes me furious when he says that" or "The kids drove me nuts today." This, however, is not the case. The true emotional triggers are not in the external situation; they are in our minds. Situations in and of themselves have no meaning to us until we *appraise* them, which is the second element of stress. Through the

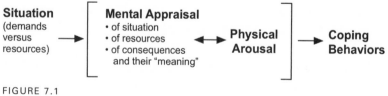

FIGURE 7.1
The nature of stress.

process of appraisal, we perceive and give meaning to situations. This evaluation process has several parts:

- First of all, we appraise the nature of the situation and the demands it is placing upon us.
- At the same time, we appraise the resources that we have to deal with it. We judge, in other words, how capable we are of coping with the situation.
- We also judge the probable consequences of coping or failing to cope with the situation and the meaning of those consequences for us.

The emotional responses that we call stress are likely to occur when we view ourselves as incapable of coping with a high-demand situation that has potentially harmful consequences for us. In response to such appraisals, our body instantaneously mobilizes itself to deal with the emergency, and we experience physiological arousal, the third element of stress. This inborn fight-or-flight response involves a general arousal of the body. Heart rate increases; breathing becomes rapid; blood pressure and muscle tension increase; perspiration may occur; and so on. All of us are familiar with the way our body becomes aroused when we perceive that we are threatened or in danger.

> The stress response includes negative thoughts, unpleasant feelings, and attempts to cope with the stressful situation.

The fourth element in our analysis of stress involves the behaviors that the person uses in order to try to cope with the demands of the situation. Responses may be mental, as when a quarterback tries to figure out which play to call, or they may be physical or social responses, such as shooting a free throw or dealing with an angry opponent.

To view this sequence in action, let us consider Kevin, who is at the plate with two outs, the bases loaded, and his team trailing by a run in the last inning. He is facing a pitcher who has struck him out twice without his even hitting a foul ball. He views the pitcher as being too tough for him (demands exceed resources). He thinks that if he strikes out again, his parents, coach, and teammates will be disappointed in him and he will be disappointed in himself. These appraisals of the situation, his ability to cope with it, and the negative consequences he expects combine to produce predictable physical results. His mouth is as dry as a ball of cotton. His legs are shaking and he can barely hold the bat. His stomach is churning, and his heart is pounding. His responses to the situation involve trying to concentrate on the pitcher and swing only at balls that are in the strike zone. Whatever the outcome of his actions, it is clear that Kevin is experiencing a high degree of stress.

Kevin's stress response to the situation seems quite natural. Most of us would probably react in much the same way. Yet some would argue that situations such as this place too much stress on children before they are psychologically equipped to handle it. Are youth sports indeed too stressful for children?

## HOW STRESSFUL ARE YOUTH SPORTS?

Researchers have used various approaches to try to measure the stressfulness of the youth sport setting. In several studies, electronic devices were attached to children so that their physiological arousal could be measured directly, through a method known as telemetry. The instruments send a radio signal to a receiver so that physiological responses, such as heart rate, can be measured while the subject is behaving normally. These studies have shown that children can experience high levels of arousal during athletic contests. For example, heart rates averaging nearly 170 beats per minute have been recorded in male Little League Baseball players while they were at bat.

The problem with this approach, however, is that physiological measures by themselves cannot tell us exactly *which* emotion is being experienced by the child. In some children elevated heart rates may reflect high levels of anxiety, while in others they may reflect simple excitement or elation. We can't tell merely by measuring the level of arousal.

To get around this problem, another approach has been to ask children to fill out rating scales of how tense, anxious, or worried they are at a particular moment. In a series of studies conducted at UCLA, Drs. Tara Scanlan and Michael Passer obtained anxiety ratings from boys and girls immediately before and after youth soccer matches. They found that most children reported rather low levels of anxiety at both points in time. However, about 20 percent of the children reported high levels of stress before the game, and many of the children reported high anxiety after games that their teams had lost.

> There is evidence that sports can be stressful,
> at least for some children.

How stressful are sports compared with other activities in which children participate? To answer this important question, Drs. Julie Simon and Rainer Martens obtained anxiety ratings from 9- to 14-year-old boys before a number of different activities, including various individual and team sports, school tests, and playing an instrument in a music contest. The researchers found that none of the sports they studied aroused as much anxiety as music solos. Moreover, wrestling was the only sport that was more anxiety-arousing than classroom tests in school. Of the various sports studied, individual sports caused the highest levels of pre-event anxiety. But, like the UCLA researchers, Simon and Martens reported that some of the young athletes experienced extremely high levels of stress before competing, regardless of the sport.

Taken together, the research results suggest that sport participation is not exceedingly stressful for most children, especially in comparison with other activities in which children have their performance evaluated. But it is equally clear that the sport setting is capable of producing high levels of stress for some youngsters. If, as some authorities have emphasized, only 5 to 10 percent of the 68 million youth sport participants experience excessive stress, this would still involve a significant number of children and adolescents. Instead of finding athletic competition enjoyable and challenging, these young athletes undoubtedly endure anxiety and discomfort, which can have harmful psychological, behavioral, and health-related effects. Such youngsters could surely benefit from attempts to help them cope more effectively with the stress that threatens their enjoyment of the sport activity.

> Parents should be alert to the signs of excessive stress.

## HOW STRESS AFFECTS YOUNG ATHLETES

Fear and anxiety are the emotions that are most frequently experienced as part of the athletic stress response. These are unpleasant states that most people try to avoid. There is evidence that this is precisely what many stress-ridden youngsters do. As shown in figure 7.2, *avoidance* of sports is one of the ways some children escape from an activity they find threatening rather than pleasant. They might like to participate but are afraid of performing poorly or of failing to make a team, so they simply do not turn out.

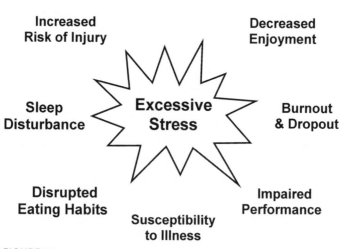

FIGURE 7.2
Negative effects of excessive stress in youth sports.

In addition to influencing decisions about entering a sport program, competitive stress can *decrease enjoyment* of sports. Instead of a challenging, fulfilling activity, sports can become a threat to self-esteem and can rob children of the pleasures they should derive from participation. This can take its toll on the athlete and produce *burnout* and eventual *dropout*. Burnout is a legitimate concern because burned-out athletes often show depression and a loss of drive and energy that carries over into other areas of their lives.

Stress affects not only how athletes feel, but also how they perform. All of us have seen athletes fall apart or "choke" under high levels of stress. When arousal is absent or extremely low, athletes frequently describe themselves as "flat" and do not perform as well as they are able. Some degree of arousal is usually needed for good performance. But at extremely high levels, arousal begins to interfere with performance. Research has shown that the more complicated or difficult the task, the less arousal it takes to interfere with performance. High-stress athletes who cannot control their emotions are likely to experience higher-than-optimal levels of arousal and to perform poorly. The failure experiences that result only serve to reinforce these athletes' fears and undermine their confidence even more. Thus, a vicious circle involving anxiety, *impaired performance*, and increased anxiety can result. In pressure situations, high-stress athletes have difficulty concentrating and thinking clearly. This also serves to interfere with performance. Many young athletes never succeed in achieving their potential in sports because of their inability to control their anxiety.

> There is an optimal level of arousal beyond
> which performance begins to suffer.

Stress can affect physical well-being as well as performance. The physical nature of the stress response taxes the resources of the body and appears to *increase susceptibility to illness* (headaches, upset stomach, or skin problems) and disease. *Loss of appetite* and *disturbed sleep patterns* also can occur. This is surely a high and unnecessary price to pay for the pursuit of athletic excellence!

Finally, research has shown that stress is related to an *increased likelihood of athletic injury.* Sports medicine specialists have also observed that athletes who find participation stressful and unpleasant often appear to take longer to recover from injuries. It may be that in some cases, an athlete finds in an injury a temporary and legitimate haven from the stress of competition.

We see, then, that stress can have many effects on athletes of all ages and that most of them are negative. Thus, athletes who develop coping skills that allow them to bear up under the pressure of competition, to be mentally tough in the face of athletic challenge and adversity, have a definite advantage.

## THE NATURE OF MENTAL TOUGHNESS

One of the highest compliments that can be paid to an athlete is to be labeled "mentally tough." Some coaches and athletes speak of mental toughness as if it were a quality that a person either has or does not have. In reality, however, mental toughness is not something we are born with; rather, it is a set of specific, learned attitudes and skills.

The specific skills that constitute what we call mental toughness fall within the brackets of the stress model described above. Mentally tough athletes mentally appraise themselves and pressure situations in ways that arouse a positive desire to achieve rather than a fear of failure. Freedom from the disruptive effects of fear of failure allows them to concentrate on the task instead of worrying about the terrible things that will happen if they fail in the situation. Another specific skill that contributes to mental toughness is the ability to keep physical arousal within manageable limits. Somehow, these athletes are able to "psych up" with enough arousal to optimize their performance without being "psyched out" by excessive arousal. What mental toughness amounts to, therefore, is specific ways of viewing the competitive situation and skills relating to self-control of emotion and concentration.

> Mental toughness is a set of specific, learnable skills.

The core of mental toughness is the ability to control emotional responses and concentrate on what has to be done in pressure situations. The mentally tough athlete is in control of his or her emotions and is calm and relaxed under fire. Such athletes do not avoid pressure; they are challenged by it. They are at their best when the pressure is on and the odds are against them. Being put to the test is not a threat, but another opportunity to achieve. Mentally tough athletes are able to concentrate on the task at hand in situations where less capable athletes lose their focus of attention. They rarely fall victim to their own or others' self-defeating thoughts and ideas, and they are not easily intimidated. Finally, they are mentally resilient and have the ability to bounce back from adversity, their determination to succeed coming across as a quiet self-assurance.

It is no accident that mentally tough athletes tend to get the most out of their physical ability. Their level of performance seems to be more consistent, and they have a tendency to perform at their best when pressure is the greatest.

> Mental toughness can give a youngster the winning edge in sports and in other life settings as well.

As a parent, you are in a position to help your young athlete develop the skills that constitute mental toughness. In doing so, you can help sport to serve as a catalyst in their personal development.

## REDUCING STRESS AND BUILDING MENTAL TOUGHNESS

### Fear of Failure: The Athlete's Worst Enemy

Aside from fears of physical injury that produce stress for some athletes, most athletic stress arises from the fact that sport is an important social situation. The athlete's performance is visible to everyone present, and it is constantly being evaluated by the athlete and by significant people in his or her life. Many athletes dread the possibility of failure and fear the disapproval of others. Some feel that their athletic performance is a reflection of their basic self-worth, and they therefore have a great need to avoid failing. They are convinced that failure will diminish them in their own eyes and in the eyes of others.

We are convinced that fear of failure is the athlete's worst enemy. The thinking of high-stress athletes is dominated by negative thoughts and worries about failing. Unchecked, these concerns with failure undermine confidence, enthusiasm, the willingness to invest and persist, and, most importantly, the athlete's belief in himself or herself. It is these thoughts that transform the competitive athletic situation from what should be a welcome challenge to a threatening and unpleasant pressure cooker. It is these thoughts that trigger the high physical arousal that interferes with performance and the ability to concentrate fully on the task at hand.

> **Fear of failure underlies most instances of "choking" under pressure.**

The ideas that underlie fear of failure do not arise in a vacuum. They almost always have been communicated to youngsters by their parents or by other important adults. This is not surprising because the basic beliefs underlying such ideas are very widespread and accepted in our culture, which emphasizes achievement as a measure of personal worth. In our society, an untold number of children fall victim to their parents' demands that they perform exactly as expected, and to condemnations when they fail. Too often, the child's achievements are viewed as an indication of the worth of his or her parents, and failure brings reprisals based on the parents' feelings that they are to blame or that they themselves are inadequate. For many children, love becomes a premium handed out on the basis of *what a child can do* rather than simply *who he or she is.*

Fear of failure is easy to create but hard to get rid of because it is reinforced by widely accepted cultural beliefs.

The fastest and easiest way to create fear of failure in a child is to punish unsuccessful performance by criticizing it or by withholding love from the youngster. Under such circumstances, children learn to dread failure because it is associated with punishment or rejection. They also learn to fear and avoid situations in which they might fail. The unfortunate lesson they learn is that their worth and lovability depend on how well they perform. Instead of trying to achieve in order to reap the built-in rewards of achievement and mastery, children strive to perform well to avoid failure. They begin to measure themselves by their performance; and if their performance is inadequate, they usually consider their total being inadequate. A child can ultimately become so fearful of failing that all attempts to succeed are abandoned. This almost guarantees that the child cannot meet the standards he or she has set, and it serves only to reinforce feelings of inadequacy.

Because they fear failure, many people never try and thereby rob themselves of opportunities to be successful.

—*John Wooden, Basketball Hall of Fame player and coach*

As a parent, you can have a dramatic impact in helping your young athlete develop a positive desire to achieve rather than a fear of failure. Earlier, we described four elements in the stress cycle: (a) the situation, (b) mental appraisal of the situation, (c) physical arousal, and (d) coping behaviors. Efforts to reduce stress and build mental toughness can be directed at all four of these elements.

### Reducing Situational Stress

The first way you can reduce stress is to change aspects of the situation that place unnecessary demands on young athletes. We are all well aware that coaches and parents can create stress by their actions. Many young athletes experience unnecessary stress because adults put undue pressure on them to perform well. Coaches who are punishing and abusive to children can create a very stressful and unpleasant environment. Similarly, parents who yell at their children during competitions or withdraw their love if the young athlete lets them down can create a situation in which the youngster "runs scared" much of the time. Eliminating such actions by coaches and parents can reduce unnecessary stress.

> Coaches can be either a source of stress
> or a buffer against its harmful effects.

Coaches enter into the life of a child for a limited period of time. But they occupy a central and critical role in youth sports and greatly influence the outcome of participation. Because of their key position, much of our research has focused on the psychological relationship between coaches and their athletes. In more than 35 years of research, we developed a series of behavioral guidelines that proved effective in helping coaches to establish an enjoyable athletic environment. The guidelines are simply a set of principles that increase the ability to positively influence others, and they can help to reduce stress.

The coaching approach described in Chapter 8 is specifically designed to counteract the conditions that create fear of failure. The same is true of the philosophy of winning discussed in Chapter 2. When coaches promote this philosophy of winning and use the behavioral guidelines presented in Chapter 8, they stand an excellent chance of creating a sport environment in which children can enjoy themselves, develop their skills in an atmosphere of encouragement and reinforcement, and experience positive and supportive relationships with their coach and teammates.

### Increasing the Athlete's Resources: Skills and Social Support

Stress is experienced when we perceive an imbalance between the demands of the situation and the resources that we have to cope with the demands. It follows that another approach to reducing stress is to increase the young athlete's resources. Two types of resources are very important: (a) the skills that the athlete possesses, and (b) the amount of support that the athlete receives from important people, such as the coach, teammates, and parents. Parents and coaches are in a position to influence both classes of resources.

It is quite natural to feel insecure when we don't have the skills needed to cope with a situation. Many young athletes experience this insecurity when they first begin to learn a sport. As their athletic skills increase, they become better able to deal with the demands of the athletic situation, and their stress decreases. Thus, being an effective teacher and working with your child to improve skills is one way that you can help reduce athletic stress. Here, again, we strongly recommend the approach described in Chapter 8 since we feel this is the most effective way to teach skills and create a positive learning environment. As athletes become more confident in their abilities, they see themselves as more prepared to cope with the demands of the athletic situation.

> Athletic stress can be combated by mastery
> of sport skills and by ample social support.

As a parent, you obviously are a potent source of social support for your child. But our research and studies of team-building have shown that coaches who use the mastery approach have more cohesive teams on which athletes like one another more. By using their "reinforcement power" to encourage teammates to support one another, coaches can help create a higher level of social support for all of their athletes. When a team can pull together and support one another in pressure situations, this kind of social support can help reduce the level of stress experienced by individual athletes.

### Developing Winning Attitudes toward Competition

Earlier, we noted that we use the term *stress* in two different ways. One use of the term relates to *situations* that place high demands on us.

The other refers to our *response* to such situations. The importance of this distinction becomes particularly clear when we deal with the role of mental processes in stress. There is a big difference between *pressure situations* and *feeling pressure*. Mentally tough athletes perform well in pressure situations precisely because they have eliminated the pressure. They report that, although intellectually they are aware that they are in a very tough situation, they really don't feel the pressure on the inside. There is no way to eliminate pressure *situations*; they will always be there because they are a natural part of competition. This does not mean, however, that athletes have to respond to such situations by experiencing high levels of stress and getting "psyched out."

Mentally tough competitors manage pressure well largely because they have become disciplined thinkers. Either consciously or unconsciously, they have made the connection in their own heads between what they think and how much pressure they feel during competition. They have learned (often the hard way) that thoughts like these produce pressure:

- "What if I don't do well?"
- "I can't blow it now."
- "I can't stand this pressure."
- "I'll never live it down if I lose."
- "If I miss these free throws, what will everyone say?"
- "If I don't sink this putt, I'll lose everything!"

On the other hand, mentally tough athletes think like this in pressure situations:

- "I'm going to do the best I can and let the cards fall where they may."
- "All I can do is give 100 percent. No one can do more."
- "This is supposed to be fun, and I'm going to make sure it is."
- "I don't have to put pressure on myself. All I have to do is focus on doing my job the best I know how."
- "I'm concentrating on performing, rather than winning or losing."

The first set of statements causes an athlete to react to adversity with bitterness, frustration, and anxiety. The second set of statements focuses attention where it should be—on giving maximum effort and concentrating totally on what has to be done. Pressure situations become welcome opportunities rather than dire threats for mentally tough athletes. The bottom line is that the fundamental difference between mentally tough athletes and "chokers" is the way they choose to construct the situation in their heads. Situations are not nervous, tense, or anxious—people are! The sooner you can help your child to realize that pressure comes from within and not from outside, the sooner he or she can start shutting it down.

---

When an athlete can start loving adversity, I know I've got a competitor!

—*Al McGuire, Basketball Hall of Fame coach*

---

One of the great benefits of sports as a training ground for mental toughness is that the consequences of failure are temporary and unlikely to have a long-term impact on the future of a child (as failing in school might). This places you in an ideal position to help your young athlete develop a healthy philosophy about achievement and an ability to tolerate failure and setbacks when they occur. The starting point for such training is the philosophy of winning described in Chapter 2. Great coaches develop mentally tough athletes and teams by realizing that an obsession with winning is self-defeating because it places the cart before the horse. They realize that effort should be directed not toward winning, but toward performing to the very best of the athlete's ability at the time. Doing the very best one can at any moment should always be the focus and the goal. Winning will take care of itself; the only thing that can be directly controlled is *effort*. Mental toughness arises in the realization that "I am performing against myself, not someone else. I will always be my own toughest opponent, and winning the battle with myself paves the way for winning the competition with my opponent."

Here are some specific attitudes that you can communicate to your child.

1. Sports should be fun.

Emphasize to your young athlete that sports and other activities in life are enjoyable for the playing, whether you win or lose. Athletes should be participating, first and foremost, to have fun. Try to raise your child to enjoy many activities in and of themselves so that winning is not a condition for enjoyment.

2. Anything worth achieving is rarely easy.

There is nothing disgraceful about it being a long and difficult process to master something. Becoming the best athlete one can be is not an achievement to be had merely for the asking. Practice, practice, and still more practice is needed to master any sport.

---

The dictionary is the only place that success comes before work. Hard work is the price we must pay for success.

—*Vince Lombardi, Pro Football Hall of Fame coach*

---

3. Mistakes are a necessary part of learning anything well.

Very simply, if we don't make mistakes, we probably won't learn. Emphasize to your child that mistakes, rather than being things to avoid at all costs, are stepping-stones to achievement. They give us the information we need to adjust and improve. The only true mistake is a failure to learn from our experiences.

4. Effort is what counts.

Emphasize and praise effort as well as outcome. Communicate repeatedly to your young athlete that all you ask is that he or she gives total effort. Through your actions and your words, show your child that he or she is just as important to you when trying and losing as when winning. If maximum effort is acceptable to you, it can also become acceptable to your young athlete. Above all, do not punish or withdraw love and approval when he or she doesn't perform up to expectations. It is such punishment that builds fear of failure.

5. Do not confuse worth with performance.

Help youngsters to distinguish what they *do* from what they *are*. A valuable lesson for children to learn is that they should never identify their worth as people with any particular part of themselves, such as their competence in sports, their school performance, or their physical appearance. You can further this process by demonstrating your own ability to accept your child unconditionally as a person, even when you are communicating that you don't approve of some behavior. Also, show your child that you can gracefully accept your own mistakes and failures. Show and tell your child that as a fallible human being, you can accept the fact that, despite your best efforts, you are going to occasionally bungle things. If children can learn to accept and like themselves, they will not unduly require the approval of others in order to feel worthwhile.

6. Pressure is something you put on yourself.

Help your young athlete to see competitive situations as exciting self-challenges rather than as threats. Emphasize that he or she can choose how to think about pressure situations. The above attitudes will help to develop an outlook on pressure that transforms it into a challenge and an opportunity to test himself or herself and to achieve something worthwhile.

---

The real competitor relishes the toughest situations. He doesn't have a choke level—he has an enjoyment level. He knows few players get to compete for the biggest rewards, and he loves it.

—*Johnny Majors, College Football Hall of Fame coach*

---

7. Try to like and respect sport opponents.

Some coaches and athletes think that proper motivation comes from anger or hatred for the opponent. We disagree. Sports should promote sportsmanship and an appreciation that opponents, far from being the "enemy," are fellow athletes who make it possible to compete. Hatred can only breed stress and fear. In terms of emotional arousal, fear and anger are indistinguishable patterns of physiologic responses. Thus, the arousal of anger can become the arousal of fear if things begin to go badly during competition.

---

Athletes who play in a generally relaxed environment where there's good will toward their opponents are less fearful and play better.

—*Tom Osborne, College Football Hall of Fame coach*

---

When children learn to enjoy sports for their own sake, when their goal becomes to *do their best* rather than *be the best*, and when they avoid the trap of defining their self-worth in terms of their performance or the approval of others, then their way of viewing themselves and their world is one that helps prevent stress. Such children are success-oriented rather than failure-avoidant. They strive to succeed rather than to try to avoid failure. Parents who impart these lessons to their young athletes give them a priceless gift that will benefit them in many of their endeavors in life.

### Controlling Arousal: Teaching Your Child Relaxation Skills

Without carefully examining our thought processes, we may have little awareness of the appraisals that we are making about situations that produce stress. But we are all painfully aware of the physical responses of our bodies to such appraisals. We respond to perceived threat by shifting into high gear on a physiological level. Our heartbeat becomes faster and stronger so that more oxygen can be pumped through our bloodstream to the muscles. Our muscles become tense in readiness to confront the emergency. Stress hormones pouring into our bloodstream increase our level of arousal. These and other physiological changes are experienced by us as the stirred-up state that we associate with emotion. As noted earlier, a moderate level of arousal can psych us up to perform more efficiently. On the other hand, high levels of arousal can interfere with our thought and behavior patterns.

Arousal can be controlled with relaxation training.

The ability to remain calm in a stressful situation, or at least to prevent arousal from climbing out of control, is a useful stress management skill. Many athletes have found that they can learn to prevent or control high levels of tension through training in muscle relaxation skills. Because one cannot be relaxed and tense at the same time, voluntary relaxation gives athletes the ability to turn off or tone down tension. Although it is clearly a skill and must be learned through work and practice, most people can be trained to relax.

Relaxation training actually has two benefits. The first is the ability to reduce or control the level of arousal, but the second is equally important. In the course of relaxation training, people become more sensitive to what is going on inside their bodies and are better able to detect arousal in its beginning stages. When they can detect the early warning signs of developing tension, they can plug in their coping responses at an early stage before the tension gets out of control.

We have been training athletes in relaxation skills for many years. We have found that children as young as 5 or 6 years of age can be trained in relaxation, and they can then use these skills to reduce tension and anxiety. Our experience has been that children who learn these and other stress-coping skills (such as the attitudes described earlier) show a marked increase in self-confidence and are less reluctant to tackle difficult situations.

Mastering coping skills at an early age
can benefit a child throughout life.

We now describe a training program that you can use to train your athletes (and yourself, if you wish) in relaxation skills. The approach that we describe involves training through a process of voluntarily tensing and relaxing various muscle groups. The goal is to learn voluntary relaxation skills while gaining increased sensitivity to body tension. We find that within about a week of conscientious training, most people can increase their ability to relax themselves and reduce tension.

If you wish to help your young athlete learn relaxation, we recommend that you go through the exercises on your own several times to become familiar with the procedure. Then you can easily guide your youngster through the exercises until they become familiar enough with them to practice without your help.

We recommend that the relaxation exercises be practiced at least once and preferably twice a day until they are mastered. They can be carried out in chairs or on a fairly soft floor (that is, on a carpeted floor or gym mats).

Explain to your child the reasons for relaxation training, and point out that many champion athletes have learned this skill. As you guide your youngster through the exercises, use a slow, relaxed tone of voice. Give the child plenty of time to experience the sensations, and make sure that he or she is doing the breathing part of the exercises correctly. The goal of the training is to combine relaxation, exhalation, and the mental command to relax repeatedly so that your young athlete will be able to induce relaxation by exhaling and mentally telling himself or herself to relax.

> Mentally tough athletes have the ability to relax themselves quickly, even in the heat of competition.

In our training procedure, we start by concentrating on the hands and arms; move to the legs, stomach and chest, back muscles, and neck and jaw; and finish up with the facial and scalp muscles. Here are the steps.

1. While sitting comfortably, bend your arms at the elbow. Now make a hard fist with both hands, and bend your wrists downward while simultaneously tensing the muscles of your upper arms. This will

produce a state of tension in your hands, forearms, and upper arms. Hold this tension for 5 seconds and study it carefully, then slowly let the tension out halfway while concentrating on the sensations in your arms and fingers as tension decreases. Hold the tension at the halfway point for 5 seconds, and then slowly let the tension out the rest of the way and rest your arms comfortably in your lap. Concentrate carefully on the contrast between the tension that you have just experienced and the relaxation that deepens as you voluntarily relax the muscles for an additional 10 to 15 seconds. As you breathe normally, concentrate on those muscles and give yourself the mental command to relax each time you exhale. Do this for seven to ten breaths.

If you train your young athlete, here is a sample of how you can phrase the instructions when presenting this exercise.

Do you know what uncooked spaghetti feels like? (They'll tell you hard, dry, and brittle. You can even have a piece with you to demonstrate.) That's almost what our muscles are like when we're all tensed up. You can't play sports when your muscles are like that. Now, what does cooked spaghetti feel like? Yes, it's soft and supple, like our muscles are when they're relaxed. What we're going to do is to learn to make our muscles like cooked spaghetti so we can quickly get rid of tension and play relaxed.

We're going to start out with the arms and hands. What I'd like you to do while keeping your eyes closed is to bend your arms and make a fist like this. [Demonstrate]

Now make a hard fist and tense those muscles in your arms hard. Notice the tension and the pulling throughout your arm as those muscles stretch and bunch up like rubber bands. Focus on those feelings of tension in your arms and hands. They're like uncooked spaghetti—hard and stiff.

[After 5 seconds] Now slowly begin to let that tension out halfway, and concentrate very carefully on the feeling in your arms and hands as you do that. Now hold the tension at the halfway point and notice how your arms and hands are less tense than before but that there is still tension present.

[After 5 seconds] Now slowly let the tension out all the way and just let your arms and hands become completely relaxed, just letting go and becoming more and more relaxed, feeling all the tension draining away as the muscles let go and become completely relaxed. And now, each time you breathe out, let your mind tell your body to relax, and concentrate on relaxing the muscles even more. That's good . . . just let go. Let those muscles become soft and supple, like cooked spaghetti.

2. Tense the calf and thigh muscles in your legs. You can do this by straightening out your legs hard while pointing your toes downward. Hold the tension for 5 seconds, then slowly let it out halfway. Hold the halfway point for an additional 5 seconds, and then slowly let the tension out all the way and concentrate on relaxing the muscles as completely as possible. Again, pay careful attention to the feelings of tension and relaxation as they develop. Finish by giving the muscles the mental command "Relax" each time you exhale (seven to ten times), and concentrate on relaxing them as deeply as possible.

3. Press the palms of your hands in front of your chest so as to tense the chest and shoulder muscles. At the same time, tense your stomach muscles hard. As before, hold the tension for 5 seconds, then slowly let the tension out halfway and focus on the decreasing levels of tension as you do so. Hold again for 5 seconds at the halfway point and then slowly let the tension out completely. Again, do the breathing procedure with the mental command to deepen the relaxation in your stomach, chest, and shoulder muscles.

4. Arch your back and push your shoulders back as far as possible to tense your upper and lower back muscles. (Be careful not to tense these muscles too hard.) Repeat the standard procedure of slowly releasing the tension halfway, then all the way. Finish by doing the breathing exercise and mental command as you relax your back muscles as deeply as possible.

5. Tense your neck and jaw muscles by thrusting your jaw outward and drawing the corners of your mouth back. Release the tension slowly

to the halfway point, hold for 5 seconds there, and then slowly release the tension in these muscles all the way. Let your head droop
into a comfortable position and your jaw slacken as you concentrate
on totally relaxing these muscles with your breathing exercise and
mental command. (You can also tense your neck muscles in other
ways, such as bending your neck forward, backward, or to one side.
Experiment to find out the way that's best for you. Tense your jaw
at the same time.)

6. While sitting in a totally relaxed position, take a series of short in-
   halations, about one per second, until your chest is filled and tense.
   Hold for about 5 seconds, then exhale slowly while thinking silently
   to yourself, "Relax." Most people can produce a deeply relaxed state
   by doing this. Repeat this exercise three times.

7. Finish off your relaxation practice by concentrating on breathing
   comfortably into your abdomen (rather than into your chest area).
   Simply let your stomach fill with air as you inhale, and deepen your
   relaxation as you exhale. Abdominal breathing is far more relaxing
   than breathing into the chest.

As you guide your young athlete through the exercises, you can practice them yourself. You will find relaxation very useful in your own life.
It not only serves as a weapon against tension and stress, but it produces
an enjoyable state in its own right.

Urge your child to use relaxation skills whenever he or she begins
to feel unduly tense. Relaxation can also be used for preparing to deal
with stressful situations by imagining these situations while concentrating on remaining completely relaxed. For example, the young athlete might imagine shooting a crucial free throw in a basketball game
as vividly as possible while maintaining as deep a state of relaxation
as possible. Relaxation together with mental rehearsal is a technique
used by many champion athletes as part of their mental preparations
for stressful athletic situations. We have found that child athletes can
also benefit from this procedure.

The stresses of athletic competition must be faced by all athletes, young and old. As a parent, you can use these stresses as opportunities to teach your youngster coping skills that will be beneficial not only in sports but in other areas of life as well. The athlete's greatest enemy is fear of failure, and anything that you can do to prevent this from developing or to teach your youngster to master it will help to make sport participation more enjoyable and productive.

# What? You Want Me to Coach?

Gregg looked stunned as he turned off his cell phone. "I don't believe what I just did."

"What was that all about?" asked his wife, Taylor.

"That was Bill Evans, the coaching coordinator of the softball league that Angie plays in. He called with this hard-luck story about how they're short of coaches and that they're considering reducing the number of teams this year. I knew what was coming when he said that Angie's been playing for three years now and that he's seen us at a lot of games. Well, to make a long story short, I let him talk me into coaching one of the teams. I can see why Bill's insurance business is so successful. Now what am I going to do? I've never coached fifteen kids before and don't know where to begin."

Taylor laughed. "It looks like you're in for a long season."

"You won't be so amused when I tell you the rest. The team also needs an assistant coach and Bill said you'd be perfect. So you're it!"

Is this scene straight out of one of your nightmares? What would you do in Gregg and Taylor's place? The fact is that many volunteer coaches become involved in precisely this way and have the same reservations about their abilities to coach. But programs could not exist without adults who are willing to devote their time and energies to coaching.

## COACHES ARE VERY IMPORTANT PEOPLE

If you are a coach, you are one of the millions of adults who make it possible for youngsters to participate in an activity that probably enriched your own life as you grew up. As we stated in Chapter 7, coaches occupy a central and critical role in the youth sport setting. Because of this, the nature of the relationship between coach and athlete is a primary determinant of the ways sport participation ultimately affects the lives of athletes. Not only do coaches occupy a key position in sports, but their influence can extend into other areas of youngsters' lives as well. For the many children from single-parent families, coaches may occupy the role of substitute parent, with enormous potential for a positive impact. The manner in which coaches structure the athletic situation, the goal priorities they establish, and the way in which they relate to their athletes can greatly influence the outcome of participation. Coaches should never underestimate their importance in the lives of their young athletes.

> A coach can be completely unaware of the
> huge influence that he or she is having.

If you are not a coach, do you have aspirations to become one? Why not seriously consider devoting some of your time and energy to this very worthwhile activity? Many potential coaches hesitate to volunteer. They think they don't know enough, or they have never been star athletes. This is understandable. Most people tend to shy away from things for which they have little training or experience. However, if you truly want to, you can acquire the necessary knowledge and skills to become a successful coach and an important person in the lives of some young athletes. Your contributions will be appreciated.

If you are not a coach and don't wish to become one, *don't skip this chapter*! The information that follows concerns basic psychological principles for any leadership role, including parenting. Additionally, knowledge of these principles will help you to evaluate the coaches in any sport program your child might participate in.

## ORIENTATION TO THE PSYCHOLOGY OF COACHING: THE MASTERY APPROACH

This chapter does not deal with technical aspects of analyzing or performing sport skills. There is an abundance of instructional material (books and videos) on teaching techniques and strategies for various sports. Also, coaching clinics that focus on sport skills and training programs for athletes are readily available. But a qualified coach must understand more than the mechanics of sports. He or she must be able to create a healthy psychological environment for young athletes—an environment that fosters athletic, personal, and social development.

In your role as a coach, you are trying to influence the behavior of athletes in desirable ways. That's where psychology, the science of mind and behavior, comes in. Simply stated, the psychology of coaching is nothing more than a set of principles that guides your behavior as a coach. Many of these principles will be recognized as things with which you are already familiar. There is nothing mystical about them. In fact, it is often said that psychology is the application of common sense. These guidelines make good sense. The challenging part comes not so much in learning the principles, but in adapting them to your personal style.

There are two basic approaches to influencing people, both of which are used by coaches. The *positive approach* is designed to increase desirable behaviors by motivating athletes to perform them and by rewarding (reinforcing) the athletes when they do. This "relationship style" goes hand in hand with the healthy philosophy of winning presented in Chapter 2. And it creates a mastery-based climate, so we will refer to it as the *mastery approach*.

The *negative approach*, which is often present in an ego-based climate, involves attempts to eliminate athletes' mistakes through the use of punishment and criticism. The motivating factor in this "command style" is fear. Punitive coaching behaviors have many undesirable side effects that can actually interfere with what a coach is trying to accomplish. It is the fastest way to instill fear of failure and to create resentment and hostility.

Both of the coaching styles are used at all levels of competition. However, the effectiveness of the mastery approach has been *scientifically validated*. This means that we are not "shooting from the hip" with personal beliefs or so-called armchair psychology about what we think will work. Rather, the behavioral guidelines (leadership principles) constituting the mastery approach were derived from our research on how coaching behaviors actually affect young athletes. The guidelines were also evaluated in numerous studies conducted in real-life sport settings. In these studies, groups of coaches were randomly placed in either an *experimental* (training) condition, in which they learned the guidelines, or a *control* condition where training did not occur. Athletes' attitudes and psychological characteristics were measured at the beginning and end of the season so that the effects of the training and control conditions could be compared. The results consistently confirmed that the mastery approach to coaching produces the following outcomes:

- fosters positive coach-athlete relations and greater mutual respect
- increases the amount of fun that athletes experience
- creates greater team cohesion and a more supportive athletic setting
- promotes higher mastery-oriented achievement goals in sports and in school
- increases athletes' self-esteem
- reduces performance-destroying anxiety and fear of failure
- decreases athlete dropout rates from approximately 30 percent to 5 percent
- produces equally positive effects on boys' and girls' teams

It's not surprising that prominent coaches recognize and practice the power of the mastery approach.

---

I try never to plant a negative seed. I try to make every comment a positive comment. There's a lot of scientific evidence to support positive management.

—*Jimmy Johnson, former National Football League coach*

---

There are three important points to emphasize about the leadership principles that constitute the mastery approach. First, they are *not sport specific*, which means they can be applied in all sports. Second, they are *not age specific*, so they can be used across all levels of competition. Third, they are *not restricted to use in sports*. For example, because parenting is a form of leadership, you can use the principles in raising your children. We now present the mastery approach behavioral guidelines.

## REACTIVE COACHING BEHAVIORS
Reactive coaching behaviors occur immediately after individual athlete or team behaviors. They include responses to (a) desirable performance and effort, (b) mistakes, (c) misbehaviors by athletes, and (d) violations of team rules.

### Reacting to Good Plays and Effort
Our concern with influencing athletes' behavior in a desirable way involves the process of learning. It is well known that people tend to repeat behaviors that produce pleasant outcomes. In this context, reinforcement refers to any event occurring after a behavior that increases the likelihood that the behavior will occur again in the future. (It is similar to the more familiar concept of reward, but psychologists prefer the term *reinforcement* because what is "rewarding" for one person may not be a reward for another.) The cornerstone of the mastery approach to coaching is the skilled use of reinforcement to increase athletic motivation and to strengthen desired behaviors.

> The most effective way to build desirable behaviors is to use your "reinforcement power."

Choosing a reinforcer is not usually difficult. But in some cases, your creativity and sensitivity to the needs of individual athletes might be tested. Potential reinforcers include social behaviors such as verbal praise, nonverbal signs such as smiles or applause, and acceptable forms of physical contact such as a high five or a fist bump. They also include the opportunity to engage in certain activities (such as extra batting practice) or to play with a particular piece of equipment.

Social reinforcers are most frequently employed in athletics. But even here you must decide what is most likely to be effective with each athlete. One athlete might find praise given in the presence of others highly reinforcing, whereas another might find it embarrassing.

> The best way to find an effective reinforcer
> is to get to know each athlete's likes and dislikes.

In some instances you may elect to praise an entire unit or group of athletes. At other times, reinforcement may be directed at one athlete. If at all possible, it is a good idea to use a variety of reinforcers and vary what you say and do so that you do not begin to sound like a broken record. In the final analysis, the acid test of your choice of reinforcer is whether it affects behavior in the desired manner.

Here are some principles for the effective use of your "reinforcement power."

1. Be liberal with reinforcement.

In our research, the single most important difference between coaches to whom athletes responded most favorably and those they evaluated least favorably was the frequency with which coaches reinforced desirable behaviors. You can increase the effectiveness of verbal reinforcement by combining it with a specific description of the desirable behavior that the athlete just performed. For example, you might say, "Way to go, Casey! You kept your head in there on the follow-through." In this way, you combine the power of the reinforcement with an instructional reminder of what the athlete should do. It also cues the athlete about what to concentrate on.

Reinforcement should not be restricted to the learning and performance of sport skills. Rather, it should also be liberally applied to strengthen desirable psychosocial behaviors (e.g., teamwork, leadership, sportsmanship). Look for positive things and reinforce them, and you will see them increase. Reinforce the little things that others might not notice. We are not promoting a sickeningly sweet approach with which there is a danger of being phony and losing credibility. When sincerely given, reinforcement does not spoil youngsters; it gives them something to strive for. Remember, whether athletes show it or not, the reinforcement you give them helps strengthen the good feelings they have about themselves.

2. Have realistic expectations and consistently reinforce achievement.

Gear your expectations to individual ability levels. For some athletes, merely running up and down the field or court without tripping is a significant accomplishment worthy of praise. For those who are more skilled, set your expectations at appropriately higher levels.

> Successful coaching requires skillful use of reinforcement.

In many instances, complex skills can be broken down into their component subskills. You can then concentrate on one of these subskills at a time until it is mastered. For example, a football coach might choose to concentrate entirely on the pattern run by a pass receiver with no concern about whether or not the pass is completed. This is where your knowledge of the sport and of the mastery levels of your individual athletes is crucial. Athletes can enjoy lots of support and reinforcement long before they have completely mastered the entire skill, if you are attentive to their instructional needs and progress.

Start with what the athlete is currently capable of doing and then gradually require more and more of the athlete before reinforcement is given. It is important that the shift in demands be realistic and that the steps be small enough so that the athlete can master them and be reinforced. Used correctly, progressive reinforcement is one of the most powerful of all the positive control techniques.

Once skills are well learned, gradually shift your reinforcement to a partial schedule. This means that some correct responses are reinforced, and some are not. Research has shown that behaviors reinforced on partial schedules persist much longer in the absence of reinforcement than do actions that have been reinforced only on a continuous schedule. As casino owners are well aware, people will put a great many coins into slot machines, which operate on partial schedules. In contrast, they are unlikely to persist long in putting coins into soft drink machines that do not deliver. Thus, the key is to start with continuous reinforcement until the skill is mastered. Then shift gradually to partial reinforcement to maintain a high level of motivation and performance.

3. Give reinforcement for desirable behavior as soon as it occurs.

The timing of reinforcement is another important consideration. Other things being equal, the sooner reinforcement occurs after a response, the stronger are its effects. Thus, whenever possible, try to reinforce a desired behavior as soon as it occurs. If this is not possible, however, try to find an opportunity to praise the athlete later on.

4. Reinforce effort as much as results.

This guideline has direct relevance to developing a healthy philosophy of winning. To put this philosophy into practice, tell your athletes that their efforts are valued and appreciated, and back up your words with action (i.e., reinforcement). Athletes' efforts should not be ignored.

---

**Don't take athletes' effort for granted.**

---

Coaches have a right to demand total effort. And this is perhaps the most important thing of all to reinforce. We stated earlier (Chapter 2) that athletes have complete control over how much effort they make, but they have only limited control over the outcome of their efforts. By looking for and reinforcing athletes' efforts, you can encourage them to continue or increase their output.

### Reacting to Mistakes

Many athletes are motivated to achieve because of a positive desire to succeed. They appear to welcome and peak under pressure. Unfortunately, many others are motivated primarily by fear of failure, and consequently they dread critical situations and the possibility of failure and disapproval. As we emphasized in Chapter 7, fear of failure is an athlete's worst enemy. It can harm performance, and it reduces the enjoyment of competing. The way you react to athletes' mistakes plays a major role in either creating or combating fear of failure.

> If managed correctly, mistakes can be
> golden opportunities to improve performance.

A typical attitude about mistakes is that they are totally bad and must be avoided at all costs. Rather than focusing on the negative aspects of mistakes, recognize not only that they are unavoidable, but that they have a positive side as well. Coach John Wooden referred to mistakes as the "stepping-stones to achievement." They provide information that is needed to improve performance. By communicating this concept to athletes in word and action, you can help them accept and learn from their mistakes.

In addition, remember that what you say and do has an important effect on athletes. Thus, deal honestly and openly with your own mistakes. When you have the confidence and courage to admit that you made a mistake, you provide a valuable role model. Such a model is important for developing a sense of tolerance for human error and for reducing fear of failure. Remember, the mastery approach is designed to create a positive motive to achieve rather than a fear of failure.

---

You must know quite well that you are not perfect, that you're going to make mistakes. But you must not be afraid of making mistakes or you won't do anything, and that's the greatest mistake of all. We must have initiative and act and know that we're going to fail at times, for failure will only make us stronger if we accept it properly.

—*John Wooden, Basketball Hall of Fame player and coach*

---

1. Give encouragement immediately after a mistake.

Athletes know when they make a poor play and often feel embarrassed about it. This is the time they are in most need of your encouragement and support.

2. If an athlete knows how to correct the mistake, encouragement alone is sufficient.

Telling an athlete what he or she already knows may be more irritating than helpful. Do not overload athletes with unnecessary input. If you are not sure if the athlete knows how to correct the mistake, ask the athlete for confirmation.

3. When appropriate, give corrective instruction after a mistake, but always do so in an encouraging and positive way.

In line with the mastery approach, mistakes can be excellent opportunities to provide technical instruction. There are three keys to giving such instruction:

- Know *what* to do—the technical aspects of correcting performance.
- Know *how* to do it—the teaching-learning approach.
- Know *when* to do it—timing.

Most athletes respond best to immediate correction, and instruction is particularly meaningful at that time. However, some athletes respond much better to instruction if you wait for some time after the mistake. Because of individual differences, such athletes are more receptive to your instruction when it is given later.

> In giving corrective instruction, don't focus on the mistake
> but emphasize the good things that will happen
> if the athlete follows your instruction.

When correcting mistakes, a three-part teaching approach is recommended. In the following example, a football player has dropped a pass because he took his eyes off the ball:

- Start with a *compliment*; find something the athlete did correctly ("Way to hustle. You really ran a good pattern!"). This is intended to reinforce a desirable behavior and create an open attitude on the part of the athlete.
- Give the *future-oriented instruction* ("If you follow the ball all the way into your hands, you'll catch those just like a pro does."). Emphasize the desired *future* outcome rather than the negative one that just occurred.
- End with another *positive statement* ("Hang in there. You're going to get even better if you work at it."). This "sandwich approach" (two positive communications wrapped around the instruction) is designed to make the athlete positively self-motivated to perform correctly rather than negatively motivated to avoid failure and disapproval.

4. Don't punish when things go wrong.

Punishment is any consequence that decreases the future occurrence of a behavior. Punishment can be administered in either of two forms: (a) by doing something aversive, such as painful physical contact or verbal abuse, and (b) by taking something that is valued away from the athlete, or more technically, by removing positive reinforcers that are usually available to an individual, such as privileges, social interactions, or possessions. With respect to the first form, punishment is not just yelling at athletes. It can be any form of disapproval, including tone of voice or action. Constant use of such punishment leads to resentment of the coach and is a probable factor contributing to lack of enjoyment and athletic dropout.

5. Don't give corrective instruction in a hostile or punitive way.

Although a coach may have good intentions in giving instruction, this kind of negative communication is more likely to increase frustration and create resentment than to improve performance.

Does this mean that you should avoid all criticism and punishment? Certainly not! Sometimes, these behaviors are necessary for instructional or disciplinary purposes. But they should be used sparingly. If you feel that you must use punishment, do it only as a last resort, and do it in such a way that it's clear that you dislike the *behavior*, not the person. The negative approach should *never* be the primary approach to athletes.

Although abusive coaches may enjoy success and may even be admired by some of their athletes, they run the risk of losing other athletes who could contribute to the team's success and who could profit personally from an athletic experience. Coaches who succeed through the use of punishment and intimidation usually do so because (a) they are also able to communicate caring for their athletes as people, so that the abuse is not "taken personally," (b) they have very talented athletes, and/or (c) they are such skilled teachers and strategists that these abilities override their negative behaviors. In other words, such coaches win *in spite of*, not because of, the negative approach.

### Maintaining Order and Discipline

Problems of athlete misbehavior during practices and competitions (games, matches, meets) can indeed become serious. In dealing effectively with this, recognize that youngsters want clearly defined limits and structure. They do not like unpredictability and inconsistency. On the other hand, they do not like it when you play the role of a policeman or enforcer. Thus, the objective is to structure the situation so that you can teach discipline without having to constantly read the riot act to keep things under control. The statements below are guidelines to maintaining order and discipline.

1. Maintain order by establishing clear expectations and a "team rule" concept.

2. Involve athletes in forming behavioral guidelines and work to build team unity in achieving them.

3. Strive to achieve a balance between freedom and structure.

These guidelines promote a cooperative approach to leadership in that athletes are given a share of the responsibility for determining their own governance. The rationale for this approach is that people are more willing to live by rules when they have a hand in forming them and

WHAT? YOU WANT ME TO COACH?

when they have made a public commitment to follow them. There is considerable research support for this rationale in psychology.

Team rules should be developed early in the season. In helping athletes to share responsibility for forming rules, use the following four-part procedure:

- Explain why team rules are necessary: "Rules and regulations are an important part of the game. If we have team rules, they will keep things organized and efficient. This will increase our chances of achieving individual and team goals."
- Explain why the team rules should be something that they can agree on as a group: "The rules will be *your* rules, and it will be *your* responsibility to follow them."
- Solicit suggestions and ideas, and listen to what athletes say to show that their ideas and feelings are valued: "What are the rules that you want to have?"
- Incorporate athletes' input into a reasonable set of rules. Rules should provide structure and yet not be too rigid. The following are examples of such rules: (a) Be prepared and focused during practice and competition. (b) Give maximum effort at all times. (c) Treat others like you want to be treated.

In addition to formulating a set of team rules, be sure to discuss the kinds of penalties that you will use for breaking them. Here again, athletes should participate in determining the consequences that will follow rule violations. And, of course, your role includes ensuring that the consequences are realistic.

Teaching self-discipline is an important youth sport objective.

The advantage of this approach is that it places the responsibility where it belongs—on the athletes themselves. In this way, team discipline can help develop self-discipline. Then, when someone breaks a team rule, it is not the individual versus *your* rules, but the breaking of *their own* rules.

4. Emphasize that during competition, all members of the team are part of it, even those on the bench.

This rule can play an important role in building team cohesion and mutual support among teammates.

5. Use reinforcement to strengthen team participation and unity.

By strengthening desirable behaviors, you can help prevent misbehaviors from occurring. In other words, you can prevent misbehaviors by using the mastery approach to strengthen their opposites. Similarly, instances of teamwork and of athletes' support and encouragement of each other should be acknowledged and reinforced whenever possible. This not only strengthens these desirable behaviors, but also creates an atmosphere in which you yourself are serving as a positive model by supporting them.

> Taking the time to develop team rules
> is easier than dealing with violations.

### Dealing with Team Rule Violations

When you have team rules, you can expect that they will be broken from time to time. As youngsters establish independence and personal identity, part of the process involves testing the limits imposed by adult authority figures—people like you! Because this is a very natural process in development, you should not feel persecuted or take it too personally. It happens with all youth coaches (as well as college and professional coaches), and therefore these recommendations for dealing with team rules are presented.

1. Allow the athlete to explain his or her actions.

There may be a reasonable cause for what the athlete did or did not do, and lines of communication should be kept open.

2. Be consistent and impartial.

In other words, avoid showing favoritism by treating *all* athletes—the stars and the subs—equally and fairly. Fairness builds respect.

3. Don't express anger and a punitive attitude.

And, of course, never take action for the purpose of retaliating.

4. Don't lecture or embarrass the athlete.

It simply is not necessary or beneficial.

5. Focus on the fact that a team policy has been broken, placing the responsibility on the athlete.

This should be done without degrading the individual or making the athlete feel he or she is in your "doghouse." Remind the athlete that a rule that he or she agreed to follow was violated and because of that a penalty must be paid. This focuses the responsibility where it belongs—on the athlete—and helps build a sense of personal accountability.

> A penalty must be paid for violating a rule
> that the team, not the coach, established.

6. When giving penalties, it is best to deprive athletes of something they value.

For example, participation can be temporarily suspended by having the player sit off to the side ("time-out" or "penalty box"). Taking away playing time or a starting position is also an effective penalty.

7. Don't use physical measures that could become aversive by being used to punish (e.g., running laps, doing push-ups).

It is not educationally sound to have beneficial physical activities become unpleasant because they have been used as punishment.

---

Children cry out for discipline, not punishment. With punishment, it's very difficult to get results.

—*John Wooden, Basketball Hall of Fame player and coach*

## SPONTANEOUS/SELF-INITIATED COACHING BEHAVIORS

### Getting Positive Things to Happen

1. Set a good example of behavior.

Children learn a great deal by watching and imitating others. Imitation (or modeling) is an important form of learning. Most athletes will have a high regard for you, and consequently they are likely to copy your behaviors and deal with sport situations in similar ways. Athletes probably learn as much from what you *do* as from what you *say*! Because of this, it is important that you portray a role model worthy of respect from athletes, officials, parents, and other coaches as well.

---

A careful man I want to be,
A little fellow follows me.
I do not dare to go astray,
For fear he'll go the selfsame way.

—*Rev. Claude Wisdom White, Sr., author/poet*

---

2. Encourage effort; don't demand results.

This is another mastery approach guideline that applies to the healthy philosophy of winning presented in Chapter 2. Most young athletes are already motivated to develop their skills and play well. By appropriate use of encouragement, you can help to increase their natural enthusiasm. If, however, youngsters are encouraged to strive for unrealistic standards of achievement, they may feel like failures when they do not reach the goals. Therefore, it is important to base your encouragement on reasonable expectations. Again, emphasizing effort rather than outcome can help avoid problems. This concept is illustrated in the words of John Wooden:

> You cannot find a player who ever played for me at UCLA that can tell you that he ever heard me mention "winning" a basketball game. He might say I inferred a little here and there, but I never mentioned winning. Yet the last thing that I told my players, just prior to tip-off, before

we would go on the floor was, "When the game is over, I want your head up—and I know of only one way for your head to be up—and that's for you to know that you did your best. . . . This means to do the best you can do. That's the best; no one can do more. . . . You made that effort."

3. In giving encouragement, be selective so that it is meaningful.
In other words, be supportive without acting like a cheerleader.

4. Never give encouragement or instruction in a sarcastic or degrading manner.
For example, "Come on, gang, we're only down 37–1. Let's really come back and make it 37–2!" Even if you do not intend the sarcasm to be harmful, youngsters sometimes do not understand the meaning of this type of communication. They may think that you are amusing others at their expense, resulting in irritation or frustration or both.

> The mastery approach to coaching is characterized
> by liberal use of reinforcement and encouragement.

5. Encourage athletes to be supportive of each other, and reinforce them when they are.
Encouragement can become contagious and contribute to building team cohesion. Communicate the enthusiasm you feel, which then carries over to your athletes. The best way to do this is by (a) presenting an enthusiastic coaching model, and (b) reinforcing athlete behaviors that promote team unity.

### Creating a Good Learning Atmosphere

Young athletes expect their coach to help them satisfy their desire to become as skilled as possible. Therefore, you must establish your teaching role as early as possible. In doing this, emphasize the fun and learning part of sport, and let athletes know that a primary coaching goal is to help them develop their athletic potential.

There is nothing mysterious about developing a good team because coaching is nothing more than teaching. Coaches impart the techniques to the players. The better job they do, the better job the players will do.

*—John McKay, former University of Southern California and professional football coach*

During each practice or competition, be sure that every youngster gets recognized at least once. Athletes who usually get the most recognition are (a) stars, or (b) those who are causing problems. Average athletes need attention, too! A good technique is to occasionally keep a count of how often you talk with each athlete to make sure that your personal contact is being appropriately distributed.

1. Always give instructions positively.

Emphasize the good things that will happen if athletes do it right rather than focusing totally on the negative things that will occur if they don't. As stated earlier, this approach motivates athletes to make desirable things happen rather than building fear of making mistakes.

2. When giving instructions, be clear and concise.

Young athletes have a short attention span. In addition, they may not be able to understand the technical aspects of performance in great detail. Therefore, provide simple yet accurate teaching cues, using as little verbal explanation as possible.

3. Show athletes the correct technique.

Demonstrate or model skills being taught. If you cannot perform the skill correctly, use accomplished athletes for demonstration purposes. A proper teaching sequence includes the following:

- Introduce a skill with a demonstration.
- Provide an accurate but brief verbal explanation.
- Have athletes actively practice the skill.

Because of the way in which athletes respond to teaching efforts, a Chinese proverb applies: "I hear and I forget. I see and I remember. I do and I understand."

4. Be patient and don't expect or demand more than maximum effort.

Acquisition of sport skills does not occur overnight. The gradual learning process is characterized by periods of improvement alternating with times in which no progress occurs regardless of the effort expended. Not only must you be persistent, but athletes must be convinced to stick to it and continue to give their best effort.

When an athlete has had a poor practice or a rough competition, the youngster should not go home feeling bad. He or she should get some kind of support from you—a pat on the back, a kind word ("Hey, we're going to work that out. I know what you're going through, but everyone has an off day sometimes."). Athletes should not leave feeling detached from you or feeling like a "loser."

5. Reinforce effort and progress.

Again, the foundation of the mastery approach is the administration of reinforcement for effort as well as desirable motor performance and psychosocial behavior.

## GAINING ATHLETES' RESPECT

All of what we have emphasized up to now is relevant to gaining the respect of athletes. There are two keys to gaining such respect:

- Show athletes that you can teach them to develop their skills and that you are willing to make the effort to do so.
- Be a fair and considerate leader. Show athletes that you care about them as individuals and that you are glad to be coaching them.

Treat athletes like they are your family. Your program discipline breeds self-discipline. Love—find something in each player to love them for. Don't spoil them—no special deals or star treatment.

—*Don James, College Football Hall of Fame coach*

Set a good example by showing respect for yourself, for them, and for others—opponents, parents, officials. You cannot demand respect. True respect must be earned.

## COMMUNICATING EFFECTIVELY

Everything we do communicates something to others. Because of this, develop the habit of asking yourself (and, at times, your athletes) how your actions are being interpreted. You can then evaluate whether you are communicating what you intend to.

> Constantly ask yourself what has been communicated to athletes and whether the communication is effective.

Effective communication is a two-way street. By keeping the lines of interaction open, you can be more aware of opportunities to have a positive impact on athletes. Fostering two-way communication does not mean that athletes are free to be disrespectful toward you. Rather, it invites athletes to express their views (both positive and negative) with the assurance that they will be heard by you. Furthermore, by presenting a model of an attentive listener, you can hopefully improve the listening skills of your athletes.

Effective communication also requires that you view a team as a group of individuals and respond to these individuals accordingly. For example, a youngster who has low self-confidence may be crushed (or positively affected) by something that has no impact whatever on an athlete with high self-esteem. By improving your sensitivity to the individual needs of athletes, you can be more successful. The ability to "read" athletes and respond to their needs is characteristic of effective coaches at all levels.

## INCREASING SELF-AWARENESS

An important part of self-awareness is insight into how we behave and come across to others—knowing what we do and how others perceive what we do. One of the striking findings from our research—in which we observed and recorded actual coaching behaviors—was that coaches had very limited awareness of how frequently they behaved in various ways. The athletes' perceptions of their coaches' behaviors were actually more accurate than the self-ratings made by the coaches. Successful implementation of coaching guidelines requires an attempt to increase the coach's awareness of what he or she is doing as well as the coach's motivation to comply with the behavioral guidelines. Fortunately, awareness is something that can be increased. Two behavioral change techniques are recommended, namely, behavioral feedback and self-monitoring.

Increased awareness can help to improve your effectiveness.

### Behavioral Feedback

Try to develop procedures that will allow you to obtain feedback from your assistants. In other words, work with assistant coaches as a team and share descriptions of each others' behaviors. You can then discuss alternate ways of dealing with problem situations and athletes and prepare yourself for handling similar situations in the future. Obviously, this requires an open relationship between coaches, a willingness to exchange feedback that may not always be positive, and a sincere desire to improve the ways in which you relate to athletes. Other feedback procedures include obtaining input from the athletes themselves. This will show your athletes that you are interested in their reactions and are motivated to provide the best possible experience for them.

### Self-Monitoring

Self-monitoring (observing and recording one's own behavior) involves taking some time after practices and/or competitions to evaluate your behaviors and actions. When going through this self-analysis, ask yourself what you did relative to the suggested behaviors in the mastery approach guidelines. To assist you in this procedure, the box below presents a brief form for self-monitoring of desirable coaching behaviors.

## COACH SELF-REPORT FORM

Complete this form as soon as possible after a practice or competition. Think about what you did, but also about the kinds of situations in which the actions occurred and the kinds of athletes who were involved.

1. When athletes made good plays, approximately what percent of the time they occurred did you respond to good plays with REINFORCEMENT? _____ %

2. When athletes gave good effort (regardless of the outcome), what percent of the time did you respond with REINFORCEMENT? _____ %

3. About how many times did you reinforce athletes for displaying good sportsmanship, supporting teammates, and complying with team rules? _____

4. When athletes made mistakes, approximately what percent of the time did you respond with:

   A. Encouragement only _____ %

   B. Corrective instruction given in an encouraging manner _____ %

   (Sum of A plus B should not exceed 100%)

5. When athletes made mistakes, did you stress the importance of learning from them?

   _____ Yes    _____ No

6. Did you emphasize the importance of having fun while practicing or competing?

   _____ Yes    _____ No

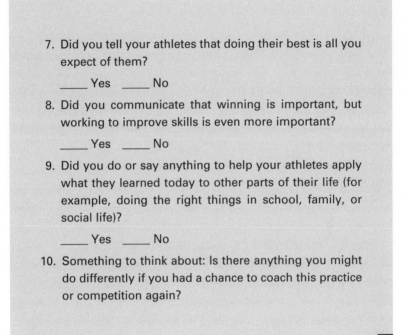

7. Did you tell your athletes that doing their best is all you expect of them?

\_\_\_\_ Yes  \_\_\_\_ No

8. Did you communicate that winning is important, but working to improve skills is even more important?

\_\_\_\_ Yes  \_\_\_\_ No

9. Did you do or say anything to help your athletes apply what they learned today to other parts of their life (for example, doing the right things in school, family, or social life)?

\_\_\_\_ Yes  \_\_\_\_ No

10. Something to think about: Is there anything you might do differently if you had a chance to coach this practice or competition again?

## COACHING YOUR CHILD CAN BE A PLUS

Coaching your own child can be a wonderful opportunity to spend quality time together, but it also presents some unique challenges for you and for your child. The most difficult issue concerns confusion arising from the dual roles of coach and parent. To effectively deal with this, you and your child need to understand that your coaching behavior and parenting behavior will be different. For example, a coach will not be able to give the immediate access or personal attention that a parent would give to a child at home. A coach must make time for all members of the team, not just one young athlete.

Four principles for the coach-parent to follow are presented below. The first two provide a foundation, which should be established in a preseason meeting with your child. The last two principles can be implemented during practices and competitions.

1. Ask your child how he or she feels about you being the coach.

In other words, get your child's perspective prior to the season. If there are reservations, it's important to discuss them. Most children enjoy playing for their parent, but some would prefer another coach. Are some kids afraid to say they would rather play for someone else? Yes, because they might believe their mother or father will feel rejected. To counteract this, you must openly communicate with your child; hear your child; encourage them to express their true feelings.

2. Discuss how your role will change when you are in the athletic environment and why you need to treat your child like any other team member.

Does the youngster feel any undue pressure, such as perceived favoritism or excessive demands from you? Many coaches tend to be harder on their child, and they bend over backward not to show favoritism. Being fair does not mean being harder on your child. It's a challenge to be impartial and treat your child no differently than anyone else on the team.

In addition to talking with your son or daughter, we recommend explaining the situation to the whole team. This can be done at the first practice or team meeting. Some coaches tell their athletes that, even though their son or daughter is on the team, they consider every athlete as one of their children. Kids are able to understand the message.

> Parent at home; coach at practices and competitions.

3. Be a mom or dad at home and a coach in sports.

Make sure your separate roles are clear in your mind and in your child's. There are at least two ways to put this principle into operation:

- Have your child refer to you as "Coach" when interacting in the sport environment. The labeling helps to solidify the separation of roles.

WHAT? YOU WANT ME TO COACH?

- If you have an assistant coach, have that person work with your child in situations involving individual instruction. If the assistant also has a child on the team, use the crisscross technique of working with each other's children.

And don't overdo it! When driving home, naturally you're going to discuss things that happened in the practice or competitive event. But set up a time interval, and don't go beyond it. Keep things in balance, and set some reasonable limits.

4. Reaffirm your love, regardless of your child's level of performance.

Youngsters will go to extremes to please their parents, and too much emphasis on sports gets things out of kilter. Above all, demonstrate in words and actions that your love does not depend on athletic ability.

Although coaching your own child may be convenient and enjoyable, you should not be the only coach your son or daughter ever has. Youngsters gain a lot by learning to adjust to other styles of leadership; thus, it is a disservice not to expose them to other coaches. Consequently, you should limit coaching your child to 2 or 3 years in a row. When the time comes to end the coaching relationship with your child, clearly explain the decision so that he or she does not feel rejected.

### SOME FINAL WORDS TO THE COACH-PARENT

As we noted earlier, scientific research has shown the beneficial effects of creating a mastery-based motivational climate. For more extensive coverage of the psychology of coaching, we recommend reading a companion book titled *Sport Psychology for Youth Coaches: Developing Champions in Sports and Life* (www.rowman.com). The principles constituting the mastery approach are also featured in a self-instructional DVD titled the *Mastery Approach to Coaching* (www.y-e-sports.com).

Youth sport coaches give a great deal of time and energy to providing worthwhile life experiences for children and adolescents. As a coach, you can increase the positive impact you have on young people's lives

by putting to use the basic principles we have described. Don't underestimate your importance in the personal and athletic development of
your athletes or the extent to which your efforts are appreciated. Strive
to make the experience as much fun and as personally meaningful for
the average and low-ability athlete as for the superstar. You will have a
lot of fun in the process.

# Male and Female High School Athletes

## *Drugs, College Recruiting, and Other Concerns*

A former All-American football player sat in the stands with his elderly father, watching his son play in a state championship football game. In the middle of the third quarter the son took the ball and ran through the opposition 82 yards for what was to be the winning touchdown. As the shouting and cheering died, the grandfather turned to his son, the former All-American player, and proclaimed, "You have now had your greatest experience in sports." Having watched his son perform similar sport heroics a generation previously, the grandfather knew whereof he spoke.

It is obviously gratifying to watch our sons and daughters perform well. They will not all win championship games; many won't make the starting team, but we hope that most school districts will provide an opportunity for all to participate. Sport participation at this age is fun and provides opportunities for self-confidence, acceptance by peers and adults, and fitness.

If sports are all that good at this age, then what are the problems? Many of the issues discussed in previous chapters apply in a special way to high school–aged athletes. We explore a few in this chapter in the hope that we may help make the high school sport experience just a little bit better.

## THE YOUNG WOMAN ATHLETE IN HIGH SCHOOL

Competing in a physically demanding activity in high school, the female athlete may encounter problems in knowing when to press ahead, when to go all out, and when to take it a bit easy. She may have relatively little understanding of how important it is to pace herself during early workouts and practices. Few things can take the joy out of sports more effectively than overexertion when one is not properly conditioned for an all-out effort.

> The need for preseason conditioning may be overlooked by the young woman athlete.

A high school female athlete should start a conditioning program with her friends before the season begins. She should be ready for that day when the coach suggests some intense efforts to see "who really wants to be on the team." Starting 6 to 8 weeks before the season to do some stretching, strengthening, and aerobic conditioning exercises with a small group of peers can be fun. It will assure them all a better chance of keeping up when they do turn out for the team.

Even in self-directed preseason exercise, the athlete may have to be reminded not to exercise when she has pain and, if some joint or tendon area begins to hurt, to ease up and give it some rest. Don't let the young woman believe that playing through pain is a smart part of sports. When it hurts you, you're hurting it!

> Academic, extracurricular, and social activities should not and need not be forgotten or sacrificed for a high school sport career.

Women's sports in high school provide opportunities of the same degree of intensity and commitment as are available to young men. Young women in high school sports can emerge as superstars, attracting all the attention and adulation that have come to select male athletes in the past. With all of this can come some exciting days for the parents and some very real responsibilities. If your household is blessed with a young woman high school superstar, be sure her sport activity doesn't unduly rule your household and everyone in it. Learn about the college recruiting process before it starts and get an unbiased appraisal by a respected college coach as to just how much potential your young athlete has in the world of collegiate sports. Most importantly, keep a close eye on those report cards and take advantage of opportunities to introduce some interest into the family life other than sports.

## Some Sport Concerns for Women Only

### Menstruation

With the marked increase in sport participation by young women, there is a very natural concern about the effect of menstruation on sport performance as well as about the impact of intense competition and training on a young woman's reproductive cycle. Research indicates that *in general*, the age of menarche (the onset of the menstrual period) is later in female athletes than in nonathletes. For example, a study of 145 Olympic athletes found that the average age of onset of menses was 13.7 years and that women athletes had a later onset than did the general population of their country of origin. Runners and gymnasts as groups had the latest onset—14.3 and 14.5 years—and swimmers had the earliest, 13.1 years. In another investigation, the onset of menstruation was found to be 14.2 years in a group of Olympic volleyball players, 13 years in high school and college athletes, and 12.2 years in a matched population of nonathletes.

The explanation for the delayed onset of maturation in athletes involves an interaction between biophysical factors (hormones and physique) and sociocultural factors. Discussion of the complex interplay is beyond the scope of this book. However, it should be emphasized that contrary to popular belief, *reduction in the level of body fat does not cause delayed menarche*!

Although menarche occurs later in athletes than in nonathletes, it has yet to be shown that exercise delays menarche in anyone.

—Dr. Robert Malina, world-renowned sport scientist

The relation of menstrual flow to sport performance has been investigated in several populations of elite athletes. Olympic gold medals have been won by women during every phase of the menstrual cycle. Elite athletes report that they train and compete without difficulty during and between periods. For whatever reason, disabling menstrual-related discomfort is less common in athletes. Dealing with menstrual discomfort in sport performance, training, and competing depends on the severity of the pain and the degree of commitment of the young woman to her sport program. A physician can prescribe medications that are quite effective in providing symptomatic relief for the discomfort experienced by many and that will permit continued training or competition. However, for a few athletes, the discomfort makes sport participation painful and unpleasant. In such cases, the young female athlete should remain on the sidelines temporarily, as it isn't necessary to prove anything by ignoring the body's signals.

Although there are fewer problems of menstrual irregularity and discomfort among athletes than nonathletes, the incidence of missed periods and the cessation of the menstrual cycle for prolonged periods occur commonly in populations of those athletes who are involved in intense training. Those young women most likely to experience missed periods and interruption of the normal menstrual cycle include (a) distance runners and other endurance athletes, (b) those making a very keen commitment to a given period of training, (c) those who had a late menarche, and (d) those who experienced irregular menstrual periods before beginning sport participation and training.

Anecdotal reports of several elite athletes who have experienced altered menstrual function with training and sport participation but normal pregnancies suggest that there is no evidence of any decreased fertility. Women athletes reportedly experience fewer complications of pregnancy, fewer Caesarean sections, shorter duration of labor, and fewer spontaneous abortions; this is not an unexpected reproductive record for a population of very fit women. For the young female athlete who is intensely involved in sport and is experiencing irregular menstrual periods, prolonged periods, or absence of menstrual cycles, a visit to the gynecologist is strongly recommended.

### Equipment Needs of the Female Athlete

With the explosion in the number of girls and women participating in sports and the great variation in the sports they are involved in, there are certain needs for better equipment for the female athlete. In most situations, female sports equipment, such as shoes, socks, shorts, pants, sweatshirts, and jerseys, is no different from that of the male athlete. All equipment should be clean and in good repair and should fit properly. This is obviously of considerable importance in regard to footwear. Proper-fitting jerseys can become important if there is underlying protective padding that must be held in place by a good-fitting jersey.

Hot weather presents a unique challenge to the woman athlete who can't go topless to expose as much heat-radiating skin as her male counterpart can. Cutoffs—half-tops exposing the lower chest and upper abdomen—are appropriate pieces of equipment for distance runners and other athletes who may train and compete in warm and humid weather.

> Attention must be given to the support and protection of the female breast in vigorous sport activities.

Being a quite freely mobile fatty structure, the female breast is not very vulnerable to significant injury. Serious bruises requiring surgery have occurred in a few rare instances in which the breasts, firmly immobilized against the chest with a wide elastic bandage, received a strong blow. With excellent breast-support bras available for the active athlete, there is no reason to support and immobilize the breasts in this inappropriate manner. There is no evidence to suggest that bumps or bruises in a well-supported breast during athletic participation will have any relation to the eventual development of cancer or tumors.

Dr. Christine Haycock, a distinguished surgeon and accomplished athlete, conducted pioneering research in the 1970s and 1980s that biomechanically analyzed breast movement of women running on treadmills. She also conducted key studies investigating breast support and protection, concluding that sports bras should have wide bottom bands for extra support and straps not so elastic that they let breasts bounce.

Along with technological advances in support, sports bras now feature welded and molded parts rather than stitched seams, which were too often the source of chafing and discomfort. And sports bras now offer high-performance moisture management. For example, Champion produces a high-support bra that combines slick nylon fabric with seamless design for "friction-free" performance, and it uses a super-wicking fiber made from coconut shells. Big brands, such as Nike, Enell, and Victoria's Secret, are also producing sport-specific bras, as styles for low-impact activities (yoga and walking) are engineered differently from those intended for running.

> As women upped the intensity of their sports, they demanded equipment equal to the task. In turn, that equipment made it possible to go longer, harder, and faster.

The female athlete may pursue sports that warrant attention to special equipment. Some sports require strength training that may involve popular pieces of equipment that have been designed for use by adult males. Young males and most females do not fit these pieces of training equipment and should use them with discretion if injuries and overuse problems are to be avoided. Also, some athletes exercise on seats designed for use by males. The dimensions of the pelvic bones on which women sit differ greatly from men's. The seats of racing or touring bicycles, of racing shells, and of white-water kayaks all may be sources of considerable discomfort to the female athlete. Seats designed for women in these sports can be specially ordered. They provide a good bit of comfort to the female and improve her performance.

### Supporting Disengagement from Intense Involvement

Prior to high school, athletics for some girls has meant an intense involvement in a variety of individual and team sports. The preadolescent and early-adolescent female willingly accepts the discipline and demanding training programs of sports and enjoys the gratifying attention of coaches and parents. As she reaches high school age, her social horizons suddenly broaden, and the young man across the aisle in homeroom isn't quite the irritation he was a year ago. Life begins to provide interesting alternatives to 5 or 6 hours a day in the gym or at the swimming pool. The young woman athlete may quite suddenly begin to underperform and put on ten pounds of fat that she can't seem to lose.

Painful as it is to accept, it is probably the end of the line. Your Olympic hopeful has had enough. Regardless of the thousands of dollars spent on lessons, fees, medical bills, and trips to competitions over the years, Mom and Dad will do well to prepare themselves to accept some new accomplishments and enjoyments of their young athlete. Some talented females who have been heavily committed to and quite successful in preadolescent sports often are disinterested in sports in high school. They may have had enough of athletics and find it a bit dull to play with less-talented, "average" high school athletes. A study of adult women who had been elite competitive swimmers as young girls found that after they left their very demanding swim programs, they shunned vigorous physical activity, and as adults they were much less active than women who had never made a serious commitment to sports as young girls.

> Be certain that the door leading out of intense sport involvement can be easily opened by a young woman athlete who has had enough.

## THE EARLY- AND LATE-MATURING MALE ATHLETE

A large number of the disappointments and problems that surround sport participation at the high school level relate to the involvement in sports by young men who are maturing at a pace that differs from the average. The implications of these maturation differences were discussed in Chapter 3 and present very real concerns in men's sports, where the ability to compete is often related to size, strength, and levels of physical maturity. Because of the special relevance of this issue to high school youngsters, the major points bear repeating here.

The early-maturing male who has experienced rapid growth in height in the sixth or seventh grade, is shaving occasionally as he starts high school, and is well-muscled before he leaves junior high school can be enjoying outstanding athletic success in youth sport programs and on junior high school teams. He has been a year or two more mature than his teammates who are of the same chronological age. During high school his teammates begin to catch up in maturation, and most will soon attain greater size and strength. No longer stronger or bigger than most of his peers, he must face what will be a painful and difficult adjustment to a less stellar role in sports. He had been a star performer because of his early physical maturity and not because of any unique skill or talent. This young man can be directed to sport participation where size and strength are not major determinants of sport proficiency, and he can be encouraged to become involved in some rewarding activities outside of athletics.

> For the early-maturing "all-star," arrange sport competition with individuals of the same maturing status rather than limiting participation to those of the same chronologic age.

Preventing high school disappointments that can be distressful for parent and athlete alike may be accomplished during the junior high school years. The outstanding eighth-grade basketball forward might work out with the high school junior varsity and thus keep his true athletic talent potential in realistic perspective. The early-maturing 14-year-old tennis champion should play some matches with the 16-year-olds to help him understand whether or not he'll continue to excel.

Frustration and disappointment of another kind is in store for the slow, delayed maturer—the young man whose growth and physical development occur after the rest of his classmates are well on their way to being physically grown-up. If the later maturer is small (and most, but not all, are), he won't be competitive in most sports because of his size. In wrestling, even though matched in competition on a weight basis, the small later maturer will not do well because of lack of strength and endurance. The small late maturer may find a positive experience in racket sports or running sports. Even if he is a tall, large, late-maturing boy, he won't have the strength or potential for endurance that will allow him to play up to expectation for someone of his size. Even in sports where strength is not a major determinant of performance, the late maturer will probably have problems due to lack of endurance.

These boys need reassurance, which is best provided by a knowledgeable health-care professional, who can inform the young man and his concerned parents about the normal progression of maturation changes and the individual's timetable for acquiring increased size and strength. If maturation is markedly delayed, an endocrinologist might be consulted regarding the possibility of endocrine treatment to hasten the maturation process.

## DRUGS AND THE HIGH SCHOOL ATHLETE

A host of drugs are available to high school students on the street and in the school. How does drug abuse relate to newly expanding sport participation by today's student population? Perhaps drug experimentation among those high school students in sport programs is little different from experimentation among the members of the student body in general. However, young men and women who have serious problems with drug abuse are not commonly found in school sports.

> The young person freaked out on drugs is not going
> to be very competitive on any sport team.

There are other reasons why the street-drug problem isn't often found in the high school locker room. Participation in a high school athletic program can provide a young man or woman athlete with a very good reason to avoid drug abuse and may give some very practical alternative highs. It puts him or her in an environment where drug abuse isn't and can't be "cool." Another reason is that drug use interferes with athletic performance, and serious abuse is readily recognized. If a troubled young athlete begins to show some unexplained changes in behavior and a real drug problem is identified, coaches and parents alike must face the issue and, in a nonjudgmental and supportive manner, get the athlete qualified, comprehensive treatment. *There are no minor drug problems among high school students.*

Although the athlete may be at less risk of abusive use of street drugs, there are a host of sport-related drug abuses that parents, athletes, and coaches must be alert to and be prepared to deal with. As we have become painfully aware, the use of performance-enhancing drugs and supplements has invaded the world of sports like never before. For parents, the scary fact is that the use of anabolic steroids (synthetic male hormones), human growth hormone, and other body-enhancing measures has begun to appear at very early levels of competition, and they are readily available to the young athlete who has the money and poor judgment to purchase them. These chemical substances are not only outlawed in sports, but many of them are known to have devastating long-term effects on the body. Lyle Alzado, a former professional football player, campaigned against the use of steroids before his death from cancer, which was attributed to steroid effects.

> Anabolic steroids will, in the long run, take their harmful toll.

Steroids are sometimes used medically in patients with certain blood disorders, severe burns, muscle-wasting diseases, and some endocrine gland abnormalities. However, studies on the long-term use of steroids have uncovered a wide variety of ill effects, including the following:

- heart disease
- sexual and reproductive disorders (e.g., atrophy of the testes, loss of libido, menstrual irregularities, infertility)
- immune deficiencies
- liver disorders (e.g., jaundice, tumors, gallstones)
- stunted growth
- psychological disturbances (e.g., violent mood swings, psychotic episodes, aggressive behavior)

Taking anabolic steroids over a long time almost invariably causes harmful effects, certainly minor ones and life-threatening effects as well. These drugs are not only dangerous but flagrantly unethical. They have no place in sports.

One of the latest fads is the use of creatine supplements, which increase the normal level of a natural body substance (testosterone) that energizes muscles. Creatine supplements allow the muscles to work longer and harder, and they have been shown to result in an increase in endurance and recovery from fatigue and the ability to train harder. The long-term effects of creatine supplements are unknown. However, most major sport organizations have expressed apprehension about their use (e.g., Major League Baseball, National Collegiate Athletic Association, National Football League). As a parent, you should be equally concerned.

It is important to counsel your youngster against the chemical "shortcuts" to strength and performance enhancement. These substances are out there and are used by even some preadolescent athletes. The glamour of athletic stardom is so great for many young people that they are vulnerable to the use of substances that may have negative effects on their future health and well-being. The strength of temptation was shown in one study in which high school athletes were asked if they would be willing to take a drug that would reduce their life span by 10 years but would also result in their ability to have a career in professional sports. The vast majority of the athletes said that they would take the drug. In today's world, the watchword is BEWARE!

## SPECIAL NUTRITION NEEDS OF THE HIGH SCHOOL ATHLETE

As young men and women begin to make their serious commitment to sport during their high school years, they encounter nutrition and training procedures designed specifically to optimize their potential for performance in a given sport. At the high school level, the most common procedures are cutting weight for participation in strength or weight-matched sports, building up (increasing body weight), and loading up on glycogen for endurance sports. All these practices can be safe when properly carried out and can contribute to the participant's success and enjoyment in the sport. The team physician, family physician, or professional nutritionist may be called upon in initiating these special nutrition practices in the young, growing athlete.

### Weight Control in Sports

Many late-maturing, small individuals are attracted to interscholastic wrestling because the competitors in this sport are matched on a weight basis, and the small size of the individual is not a handicap. In addition to small late maturers in the lower weight classes, many young men weighing 120 to 150 pounds who are too small to be competitive in football or basketball find wrestling an attractive winter sport. In fact, there is a disproportionate number of participants in the weight classes between 120 and 145 pounds, so competition for varsity positions at these weight classes may be very intense. The wrestlers often try to manipulate their weights to compete in a weight class in which they think they may have the best chance of being on the first team. This can lead to serious abuses, such as fluid restriction, starvation, and use of diuretic pills and cathartics.

> The goal for most effective participation in a
> weight-matched sport is to take into competition the
> maximum amount of strength, endurance, and quickness
> for every pound of body weight.

The athlete should go into competition with a minimum level of fatness compatible with optimal fitness. The estimated minimal-fatness level of 5 to 7 percent of body weight satisfies this goal and has been found to be the level of fatness of high-performing wrestlers and other elite athletes in weight-matched sports. It is recommended that every candidate for the wrestling team have his body fat estimated 6 to 8 weeks before the competing season begins. When the athlete knows what his fatness level is, he can calculate what his competing weight would be at 5 to 7 percent body fat. He then knows that he can be most competitive at that weight, allowing 3 to 4 pounds for growth during the season. Most candidates have excess fat that must be lost to reach their desired competing weights. This can be done by increasing their energy expenditures with after-school, preseason conditioning and by limiting their diets to no less than two thousand calories each day. The rate of fatness loss should be no greater than 2 or 3 pounds per week. Thus, it is essential to initiate the program well before the competing season. *There is no way in which fat can be reduced rapidly without sacrificing normal growth and reducing muscle.*

In certain strength-related sports, such as men's gymnastics and figure skating, fat in excess of the minimum compatible with optimal fitness will hinder performance. As in wrestling, estimating fatness and reducing it with modest diet reductions and increased energy expenditure at a carefully controlled rate will be compatible with good performance and good health.

### "Bulking Up" for Sport

Each year, hundreds of thousands of adolescents try to increase their body weight and size to increase their potential for sport performance.

In a study of 48 varsity football players in four different high schools, more than two-thirds of them had used special diets, drugs, and supplements to try to increase body weight at some time during their high school careers. The young person trying to increase body size for a sport needs professional supervision by a physician who appreciates the sincere commitment of the athlete and the importance of his or her concern with body size.

An interested physician can play a critical role in a young person's weight-gaining efforts by estimating maturity status and growth potential and recommending safe and effective methods for gain in muscle weight. The athlete must realize that only an increase in muscle mass will increase his or her potential as an athlete. Simply getting fatter will accomplish nothing and may threaten later health.

> Muscle work increases muscle size, mass, and strength. There is no hormone, vitamin, protein, or nutritional supplement that *safely* promotes this.

The athlete trying to gain weight must follow a professionally supervised weight-training program of muscle work and must ingest the increased amount of food needed to support the increased growth of new muscle. This diet should be one low in cholesterol and saturated fats, limited in salt, and high in fiber content. A diet for weight-gaining purposes in high school can be a very positive nutrition-education experience for young athletes and their families. A conscientious high school athlete can gain as much as 1 to 1.5 pounds a week with a well-supervised program and a high degree of enthusiastic compliance.

### Glycogen Loading for the Endurance Athlete

Relatively few young athletes at the high school level become involved in competitions that are positively influenced by so-called glycogen loading, or super-compensation. Long-distance cross-country skiing and marathon running are classic examples of sports in which maximizing the concentration of muscle starch—glycogen—enhances the athlete's performance. Muscle glycogen concentrations are maximized by vigorously exercising the muscles used in the sport event for 3 or 4 days while maintaining a controlled amount of carbohydrate in the diet. The resulting depletion of glycogen in the muscle stimulates muscle enzymes to overcompensate the level of glycogen that is retained in the muscle when the athlete then takes in a high-carbohydrate diet. While ingesting the high-carbohydrate diet, the athlete must reduce the intensity of the training for 4 days prior to the competition. Glycogen loading is a very demanding regime and appropriate only for seriously committed athletes in true endurance events.

## SICKNESS AND INJURY

As a group, high school athletes are the healthiest members of a very healthy segment of the population. They can, however, encounter minor illnesses brought on by nonspecific respiratory infections, such as colds and flu. To a competitive high school athlete, however, there are no such things as minor illnesses.

---

An athlete with a fever should not practice, work out, or play without a physician's examination and clearance.

---

Fever responses to illness vary considerably among individuals, but as a general rule, a fever of 100 degrees or greater should put an athlete on the sidelines. Not only will an athlete with a fever play poorly (regardless of all protests to the contrary), he or she will expose other teammates to the infection. There is also a very remote possibility of the cold or flu virus affecting heart muscle so that it won't tolerate the stress of vigorous exercise. Even the finest body can use a little help with rest in combating an infection. That will help make the illness as brief as possible.

On rare occasions, the high school–aged athlete can be laid low with something more serious than a common cold or nonspecific viral infection. Infectious mononucleosis or severe strep throat (streptococcal pharyngitis) can put the young athlete in bed for a week or more.

Coming back from such a setback can be demanding and frustrating. The athlete will need all the support and understanding he or she can get from parents, teammates, and the coach.

> **As a general rule, it will take at least 3 days of reconditioning for every day of illness and inactivity.**

The infection that keeps the basketball starter in bed at home for a week may set him back in conditioning three weeks, after he feels completely well. Getting back to training before he is completely well, free of fever, and able to go to school all day will only prolong his illness and the period of underperformance. Why the body responds in this way isn't well understood, but endurance and strength come back very slowly after a significant infection and enforced inactivity. The experience may be made a bit more tolerable if athletes know how long it is going to take to get back to pre-illness levels of performance.

The increased intensity of competition, the greater size and strength of athletes, and the greater periods of time athletes spend at sports all contribute to the increased risk of injury in high school sports. Chapter 6 is devoted to the nature and management of sport injuries. Parents should become familiar with that chapter and should share with their athletes information about how the athlete's minor injuries are to be managed at home. Together you should prepare an optimum treatment plan for minor sprains, strains, and contusions. Know how to effectively provide *ICE* treatment over the weekend to those hurts from a Friday night game. Have elastic bandages wet and refrigerated and plastic produce bags ready for crushed ice. Know how to elevate a bed to keep an injured ankle from swelling overnight. Have ice cups in your freezer to provide ice massage for minor overuse injuries that can be effectively treated during an evening.

Inadequately rehabilitated sport injuries are found throughout high school sports. Adequate rehabilitation of an injured ankle, knee, or shoulder is the greatest unmet need in the medical care of high school athletes.

A weakened leg or arm puts an athlete at increased risk to another injury and obviously hurts performance. Following an injury, an arm or leg should be exercised until the strength and range of motion of joints are equal to those of the uninjured arm or leg. This degree of rehabilitation should be reached before the athlete attempts to return to practice or competition. Getting the athlete to the rehabilitation facility, providing specific exercise needs at home, and observing your youngster's progress are important contributions by parents to injury management.

An additional aspect of injury management, and one that may seem somewhat peripheral to the injury, is the maintenance of fitness during the period of recovery from a sport injury. In addition to the obvious need to stay fit for the most prompt and effective return to competition, the high school athlete needs some sport-related activity to occupy those hours that were previously given to athletic endeavors. The young man or woman with an injured arm can run and do lower-extremity weight training. The individual with a lower-extremity injury can soon begin to swim or work on upper-body weight training. Separating a previously busy high school student-athlete 2 or more hours every afternoon from friends still involved with the team is an invitation to some less-than-desirable activities. Coaches, busy with their teams, cannot be expected to fill these hours. Encouragement and support from home will often be needed.

## PARENTS' RESPONSIBILITIES IN SPORT INJURIES

1. Be prepared for treatment at home.
2. Be sure rehabilitation is complete.
3. Encourage the athlete to stay fit.

## HOW TO HANDLE COLLEGE RECRUITING

In the early 1900s, when an Ivy League university constructed a football stadium that would seat tens of thousands of spectators, collegiate sports became big business. And, as you likely know, they have continued to be so. If your son or daughter has had a truly outstanding high school sport career, he or she is going to be invited into this multibillion-dollar enterprise. He or she will be recruited.

For the high school athlete and his or her parents, recruiting can be a very positive culmination of a fine high school athletic career. Or it can mean weeks of irritation, frustration, and anxiety, leading eventually to a much-regretted decision about the athlete's future education and athletic opportunity.

Playing the recruiting game demands a well-thought-out game plan. What follows are some guidelines to how the recruiting game is played and how to end up a winner:

- Know the rules. Don't try to play this game without knowing them.
- Know how good your athlete really is. How badly are people really going to want him or her in their program?
- Set down some guidelines and rules for dealing with recruiting in your own personal family situation. What are you going to allow and what is going to be off limits in your particular situation?
- Know as specifically as possible what your son or daughter really wants in a school. What kind of an academic program and school should it be, and where should it be located? What kind of sport program will your child be happiest in? These things should be well thought through before the recruiters are in the living room.
- Parents and athletes alike have to realize at the outset that they must be completely honest with themselves and the schools' representatives. Prolonging the attention and the courting may be a titillating game, but the athlete will end up the loser. Recruiters who are not dealt with in a reasonably straightforward way won't be misled. Your athlete isn't the first one they ever tried to entice to their school.

### How Will Colleges and Universities Know about Your High School Athlete?

Intercollegiate sport is an intensely competitive enterprise, and one can feel quite confident that little of the talent that makes for winners is ever going to be overlooked. In spite of the instances in which eventual sport stars were overlooked, true athletic talent at the high school level is not apt to be bypassed. High school coaches get great satisfaction in bringing to the attention of college coaches their "well-coached" young stars. The college coaches, their assistants, former athletes, and other alumni all monitor high school sports in various geographic areas on the lookout for the potential collegiate performer. In addition to these scouting efforts, there are highly efficient professional scouting services subscribed to by collegiate sport programs. They provide sophisticated, professional evaluations of high school athletes from all across the country. For an appropriate fee, these services give college coaches professional analyses of high school athletes that they observe in summer camps, preseason workouts, and actual competition wherever an outstanding high school athlete may perform. If your son or daughter has the potential to be a collegiate athlete, college coaches are likely to know about it.

> The first step: learn the rules of the recruiting game.

Playing any game demands that the players know and abide by rules. It is especially true in the recruiting game. Breaking the rules (and the easiest way to break the rules is not to know them) can cost your son or daughter a college athletic career and perhaps a college education. At the very first sign of college athletic recruitment, obtain a copy of the *Guide for the College-Bound Student-Athlete*—available from the National Collegiate Athletic Association (www.ncaapublications.com/productdown loads/CBSA.pdf). The young athlete and his or her parents should be familiar with the information in this 24-page pamphlet.

### How Good Is Your Athlete? How Much Interest Will Colleges Show?

It is essentially impossible for any parents to be completely objective in appraising the real abilities and talents of their children. It is hoped that most parents perceive their offspring (regardless of intermittent evidence to the contrary) as sensational. The high school coach of your talented son or daughter may also lack objectivity. Yet it is important to get a reasonable measure of the young athlete's true potential and capacity to compete. One suggestion that has served as a good technique for several high school seniors is to seek out a nearby college or junior college coach at a school in which the athlete has no recruitment interest. Make arrangements to get that coach's professional appraisal of the athlete. In this way, at least one major question can be answered: is the athlete physically big enough and quick enough to play competitively in college? Most high school competitions don't test these traits to the degree that they will be needed in college competition. The 6-foot, 6-inch high school basketball player is going to be middle height in college basketball and may be a half-step slow in the eyes of a college coach. It is best to know from the start any limitations your athlete might have and what level of college competition he or she can play at.

### Establishing Some Recruiting Ground Rules

Before things go any further, some questions about handling recruiting are in order. Who will talk to the recruiters? How are you to decide to whom to talk? Whom will you allow to visit in your home? How are you to control the effects of these invasions on your athlete's school responsibilities and after-school life? How are you going to keep some balance with other family members' interests and priorities?

Some planning can eliminate much of the disruption and potential distress. First, some decisions should be made as to what the athlete sees as top priorities in his college experience:

- How important are prestigious academic opportunities, and in what general academic areas do your athlete's interests lie?

- How competitive is he or she academically?
- Does your athlete need academic assistance?
- Does the athlete feel strongly about staying close to home, or is there a sincere desire to go to some other part of the country?
- Will your athlete go anywhere for the right academic and/or sport program?
- In what kind of sport program will the athlete be most successful and satisfied?
- What style of play, coaching, and team personality will he or she find most satisfying?

Answering these questions early in the recruiting process may eliminate a large percentage of interested schools. It is not uncommon, if they have kept in close touch with the athlete's high school coach during these discussions, for the family and athlete to have the coach screen all the interested schools and their recruiters. The coach can determine which schools satisfy the criteria developed in earlier discussions. Probably no more than a half-dozen schools will be of real interest to even the most sought-after high school star.

> Much of the harassment of outstanding athletes
> and their families during the recruiting process
> has been reduced by NCAA legislation.

No recruiting is allowed during the active sport season in high school. The athlete is restricted in the number of colleges he or she can be invited to visit, and the number of visits is also regulated. The number of home contacts is limited to three.

Visits by recruiters are followed by visits to a limited number of campuses. These visits, of course, are highly structured sales pitches carefully orchestrated to impress the student-athlete. He or she will have no problem getting to see the part of university or college life that is thought to appeal most. Students are shown the athletic facilities and they visit with the athletes—perhaps even eat at the training table—but they can spend no more than forty-eight hours at each campus visit.

Experienced coaches often gain a good deal of insight into the personality and maturity of the athlete during the on-campus visit. This social glimpse is an important part of the recruiting process for both parties. Is this big, quick athlete going to be a coachable team player? More than one young athlete has found a school's interest cooled or terminated after the on-campus visit.

The NCAA has legislation concerning high school academic-performance standards required for admission to varsity athletic programs in member colleges and universities. They are more stringent than in the past and are a sharp reminder to the talented high school athlete not to neglect high school scholastic responsibilities.

> During the all-important senior year of high school, when sport performances can be truly outstanding and a heavy responsibility, academic matters cannot be ignored.

Being a parent of a high school athlete can sometimes provide some of your greatest moments. Most certainly, it will provide some of the real challenges. Nobody ever said that being a parent of an active, growing young person was going to be dull, predictable, or easy. Remember that the goal of sports must always be, first and foremost, to have fun—for the high school participant and certainly for the parent, who can do no better than allow that high school youth to continue to grow up and away through experiences in sports.

# Surviving Youth Sports

## A Commonsense Approach to Some Challenging Issues

Before writing this book, we interviewed numerous parents, sport program administrators, coaches, and young athletes. We felt that the kinds of issues with which they were having difficulty needed to be covered. In this final chapter, we present common problems along with recommendations derived from a combination of research-based information and common sense.

### PUTTING SPORTS IN PERSPECTIVE FOR YOUR CHILD

In the preceding chapters we have shown how athletics can contribute to youngsters' personal, social, and physical well-being. Sports are an important part of life for millions of young people. And for a small number, youth sports are the first phase of a journey that ends in a career in professional athletics. Perhaps you hope that your child is headed in this direction.

---

You give up a lot of time for this stuff as a family, and there's sort of the expectation: we're going to get something out of this.

—*Mother of an outstanding high school basketball player*

---

To strive for high standards of athletic excellence is commendable. But parents and athletes alike must realize that the chances of playing college sports or of actually becoming a professional are remote. Even if your child appears to be a gifted athlete, the odds are overwhelming. In regard to this, the National Collegiate Athletic Association has compiled estimates of the probability of competing beyond the high school level. The following represent the *percent of high school athletes (a) who participate at the intercollegiate level, and (b) those who rise to the world of professional sports*:

- men's basketball      (a) 3.2%      (b) 0.03%
- women's basketball    (a) 3.6%      (b) 0.03%
- football              (a) 6.1%      (b) 0.08%
- baseball              (a) 6.6%      (b) 0.6%
- men's ice hockey      (a) 10.7%     (b) 0.1%
- men's soccer          (a) 5.7%      (b) 0.04%

> The stiff odds against a child's becoming a college or professional athlete indicate that youth sports should not be treated as a feeder system. Instead, the focus should be on personal growth and development.

Given the reality of the situation, a career in professional sports or even participation at the college level is an unrealistic goal for the vast majority of young athletes. It is therefore important to impress upon them that sports are but one part of their life. It is all too easy for youngsters and parents alike to harbor fantasies of turning pro and to sacrifice other areas of their development in pursuit of that fabled status and its rewards of fame, money, and glory. It is not at all uncommon for athletes to become one-dimensional.

Some college athletes mistakenly forsake educational opportunities, to their own later despair. They view college as only preparation for their (hopefully) professional careers in sports. Schoolwork is seen as important only to maintain athletic eligibility. As a result, such individuals fail to actually graduate. Thus, unhappily, the lofty ideal of the scholar-athlete often does not extend beyond the silver-tongued pitch of the college recruiter.

Although the problem may be most readily apparent in college, it doesn't start there. Putting young athletes on pedestals and granting them special favors may in the long run be a disservice to them. Be thankful if your youngster does have athletic ability, but at the same time help him or her to develop into a well-rounded person. As valuable as athletics can be for developing youngsters, we do not believe spiritual enrichment, social and academic development, and quality of family life should suffer. Sports can offer both fun and fulfillment, but there is more to life than sports.

Perhaps the best advice we can give is to encourage your child to participate in sports if he or she wishes to, but at the same time do not allow the tail to wag the dog. Help your child to understand that sport participation is not an end in itself, but a means of achieving various goals. Teach your child to enjoy the process of participation for itself rather than to focus on such end products as championships and college scholarships. Neither victory nor defeat should be blown out of proportion, and no parent should permit a child to define his or her self-worth purely on the basis of sport performance. By keeping sports in perspective, you can make it a source of personal and family growth.

## PROVIDING AND SUPPORTING ALTERNATIVES

The total development of the child is best served by participation in a variety of activities. Thus, part of putting sports in perspective involves encouraging and allowing your youngster to grow in a variety of directions, one of which might well be participation in sports. But there is an important instance in which sports are not an option in the child's life—when a child decides that he or she does not wish to participate.

In accordance with the "Bill of Rights for Young Athletes" presented in Chapter 1, we support the basic right of every child to participate in athletics. Sometimes, however, children make the decision not to play. When this happens, many parents are confused and disappointed, particularly if they have looked forward to their child's involvement in sports. It is hard under these circumstances to respect a child's decision, but in many cases it is very important to do so.

> If your son or daughter decides not to participate in sports, the most important first step is to *find out why.*

Tell your child that you believe it's an important part of growing up to take responsibility for one's own decisions, but that you wish to understand the reasons why he or she doesn't want to play. You need to find out whether the child's decision is based on a lack of interest in the sport or whether it is based on other considerations. For example, some children would actually like to play but decide not to because they don't have confidence in their level of ability or in their acceptance by their teammates. Thus, the most important factor is to decide whether the child would actually like to play. If so, then you as a parent may be able to reassure and encourage your child to give it a try and see how things work out. You should point out that skill levels will increase through participation and that the job of the coach is to help team members become the very best athletes they can.

Sometimes a young athlete decides not to participate because of fear that he or she might let parents down or lose their approval by not performing well enough. If this is the case, you have a golden opportunity to deepen your relationship with your child by exploring his or her feelings and clarifying your own values and expectations. You must face head-on the concern that your child has and the extent to which it is based on reality. The fear may be based on the child's realistic perception of what you expect from him or her. If so, some adjustments in your own thinking may be important. Are you willing to accept your child for what he or she is? Can you love your little benchwarmer? Can you be satisfied with your child merely striving to become the best he or she can be, not only in sports but in other activities? If so, and if you can communicate this honestly to your son or daughter, this lesson can contribute to lifelong growth.

## WHAT TO DO IF YOUR CHILD IS ELIMINATED FROM SPORTS

Heartbreak can be experienced when youngsters are eliminated from sport participation. Surely, not all children can be on the team of their choosing, but we believe that every youngster should have a chance to play. Prior to the age of 14, the practice of cutting children from sport programs is indefensible. During high school years, it is appropriate to have select leagues to allow gifted athletes to develop their skills. But even at this level, alternative programs should be available for less-talented youngsters who wish to play the sport.

The tragedy of cutting children from sport programs lies in the fact that those cut are almost always the least skilled or those who have discipline problems. It is precisely these youngsters who are in need of an opportunity to grow through sport. Here again, we must choose between a professional model and one devoted to the development of athletes. Applying the professional model is certain to lead to a lot of disappointment. As Basketball Hall of Famer Bill Russell described the world of professional sports, "Those who don't make the team get tossed out on the street. It is a very serious business." In choosing a program for your youngster, you should keep this in mind.

What should you do if your child is cut from a team? The first thing is to realize that whether or not your child shows it, he or she is likely to feel disappointed, rejected, and perhaps even humiliated. The youngster truly needs your support at this very difficult time:

- You can give support by acknowledging the disappointment felt by the child.
- Do not tell the child not to be disappointed or make unrealistic excuses for why it happened.

> All people must learn to face disappointments in life.
> You can make this easier if you show that your love
> and esteem for your child have not diminished.

In addition to communicating your understanding acceptance and providing reassurance, you can help your child become involved in other programs or other activities. Help your child to investigate options in other programs in the same sport or in other sports. One child who was at first devastated by being cut from a football team was helped by his parents to get involved in a soccer program and is now having a great time. Your child might also choose a nonathletic activity. If so, that decision should be supported.

Being cut from a team may be particularly painful at the high school level. Moreover, youngsters in this age range, particularly boys, may be unwilling to openly express the hurt they feel. Creating an atmosphere that will help him explore his feelings may help to ease his sense of rejection.

## PERFORMANCE IN SCHOOL AND PLAYING SPORTS

Should poor grades keep your child from playing sports? There is no simple answer to this question, but two varying perspectives should be considered. First, all children need vigorous physical activity as part of their daily lives, and sports provide all the benefits of exercise and the potential for acquiring a sense of accomplishment. If a child is having trouble in the classroom, sports may be an important avenue of success in his or her life, so it could be harmful to take it away. In fact, when youngsters feel a sense of success in athletics, this can enhance their self-esteem, which carries over to other areas, including academics. The second perspective emphasizes that practices and competitions can be time robbers from schoolwork. Consequently, when sports-related demands become excessive, it might be in the child's best interest to disallow participation.

What should you do if your young athlete is having trouble keeping grades up?

- Start by looking for other causes of poor classroom performance. Too much TV watching might be one problem; conflicts with other duties, such as a job, might be another cause.
- Ask your child what can be done to help him or her improve at school. Plus, input should be sought from coaches, teachers, and school counselors.
- In some cases, you and the school may decide that the young athlete is not studying enough. In this situation, it is reasonable to make sports involvement dependent upon achieving better grades.

### WHAT TO DO IF YOUR YOUNGSTER WANTS TO QUIT

At one time or another and for a variety of reasons, most athletes think about quitting. Sometimes a decision to quit comes as a shock to parents, but at other times the warning signs leading up to the decision are very clear.

What are the causes of dropping out of youth sports? In general, the reasons fall into two categories. The first category involves a shift in interests, especially in adolescents. Other involvements, such as a job, a boyfriend or girlfriend, or recreational pursuits, may leave little time for sports. In such cases, a youngster may simply choose to set other priorities.

The second category of reasons why youngsters drop out relates to negative sport experiences. Research has shown that the following reasons often underlie a decision to drop out:

- not getting enough playing time
- poor relationships with coaches or teammates
- an overemphasis on winning that creates stress and reduces fun
- over-organization, excessive repetition, and regimentation leading to boredom
- excessive fear of failure, including frustration or failure to achieve personal or team goals

If the youngster has decided that other activities are more important, his or her priorities should be respected. However, it is wise to provide a reminder that a commitment has been made to the program and to teammates. In other words, athletes owe it to themselves and to others to honor commitments and to finish out the season. This gives the youngster an opportunity to feel good about himself or herself by fulfilling the obligation through the rest of the season—even if the activity itself is no longer pleasurable.

If the decision to quit is based on one or more of the negative factors listed above, there is a legitimate cause for concern. Consequently, the situation requires open discussion to probe some ways to resolve the difficulties being experienced. As a last resort, you may wish to take some active steps to correct the difficulties. This may involve speaking to the coach or league administrators. In talking with your youngster, you should evaluate how intolerable the situation is to him or her and whether the problems can be worked out. In all but the most severe cases, you can point out that a commitment has been made, and you can encourage your youngster to finish out the season.

> It is very important to find out the reasons your child wants to quit and see if potential problems can be solved.

If the problems are sufficiently severe, the decision to drop out may be in the best interests of the child. In this case, you would want to communicate to your child that although it is important to live up to commitments, you understand that the principle is outweighed by the nature of the problems. If the child does drop out, there may be other opportunities to play in a sport program that doesn't have the negative factors that prompted the decision to quit.

## THE RISK OF EATING DISORDERS

Young athletes usually are concerned about looking good, and they all want to perform well. Most of the time, these factors motivate them to work hard at conditioning their bodies and perfecting their skills. But sometimes, to attain these goals, athletes resort to self-destructive methods that result in serious medical disorders, such as anorexia and bulimia. *Anorexia* is a type of eating disorder in which people have an obsessive fear of gaining weight. They severely limit the amount of food they eat and become dangerously thin. *Bulimia* is characterized by episodes of binge eating (consuming a large amount of food in a short time). This is followed by attempts to get rid of the food (purge) by vomiting, excessively exercising, or using medicines like laxatives.

> In some thin-build sports (e.g., figure skating, gymnastics) and in some weight-regulated sports (e.g., wrestling), the incidence of eating disorders is alarmingly high.

Various sports medicine studies report rates of eating disorders as high as 60 percent, and disorders occurring in athletes as young as 8 or 9 years of age. It is essential to recognize that such maladies are neither restricted to athletes in the sports mentioned here, nor do they only occur in females. Athletes in all sports are at risk for eating disorders.

The following are unhealthy weight-control methods that can have devastating effects on the body:

- use of diuretics (substances that cause excess water excretion)
- use of laxatives
- self-induced vomiting
- excessive and compulsive aerobic exercise
- dieting that approaches self-starvation

Because of the health-related risks, parents and coaches should be alert for the warning signs of a developing eating disorder:

- excessive preoccupation with being "fat," especially in an athlete who is normal weight

- unusual eating habits, especially signs of excessive (and often, secret) food intake (the first part of the binge-purge pattern of bulimia)
- evidence of purging with laxatives or by vomiting (one sign of repeated vomiting may be sores at the corner of the mouth or on the tongue caused by stomach acid)
- food avoidance or severe caloric restriction
- alternating periods of lethargy and irritability

If you or your child's coach detects one or more of these signs, you should talk with the youngster in a highly supportive manner. If an eating disorder is suspected or detected, professional counseling should be sought.

## HELPING YOUR CHILD INTERPRET CAUSES OF SPORT OUTCOMES

The judgments we make about the causes of events in our lives are of major importance. In understanding something that happens, we are often asked to decide how much the event was caused by us (factors within ourselves) and how much it was caused by factors outside of our control, such as chance or the actions of others. Sport experiences can be an important training ground in forming accurate causal perceptions.

As a parent, you can objectively point out what you perceive to be the cause of your child's sport experiences. This can help a youngster form a more realistic way of looking at things. As adults, we have our own biases in perception, but we can try to be as objective as possible. For example, if your child blames a loss on a bad call by an umpire or a referee, you might point out that he or she did not play up to capabilities. This helps the child evaluate his or her own role in the outcome. On the other hand, a low-self-esteem youngster who blames himself or herself for a defeat may be helped if you point out that the opponent was highly talented and played well that day.

When disappointments occur, some parents erroneously try to protect or comfort their youngsters by blaming others.

The favorite target of parents may be the coach, teammates, bad luck, or fate. In such cases, children are never faulted for failure to achieve, for it is always due to some external cause. Parents who express such attributions may be doing their children a disservice by communicating that they are never responsible for what happens to them. Such children may begin to view the causes of what happens to them as beyond their control. As a result, they may lose sight of the responsibility they have for their own behavior and its consequences.

When parents do help their children to accurately interpret the causes of events, children can develop a balanced perception of reality. This is but another way that sports can serve as a valuable arena for learning lessons and acquiring skills that can be applied throughout life. As a parent, you can participate in and foster the process.

### What to Do after a Tough Loss or During a Losing Streak

Children differ a great deal in their reactions to a loss. Some may be barely affected or may forget the loss almost immediately. Others will be virtually devastated by the loss and may be low-spirited for days. If your young athlete feels down about a loss, you should give him or her a chance to feel and express the emotion. If, for example, the youngster cries after a loss, this is a realistic expression of depth of feeling and should be accepted as such. At a time like this, a child needs parental support rather than a command to "act like a man."

Respect and acceptance of feeling demands that you not deny or distort what the child is feeling. If your daughter has struck out three times and made an error that lost the game, she does not want to hear, "You did great." She knows she didn't, and your attempts to comfort her may well come through as a lack of understanding about how she feels. Likewise, it is not very helpful to tell a child that "It doesn't matter." The fact is that at that moment it does matter a great deal!

---

**Valuable lessons can be learned from both winning and losing.**

---

One thing you can do after a loss is to point out something positive that was achieved during the competition. For example, a wrestling match may have been lost, but some good takedowns and escapes may have been executed. By emphasizing accomplishments, you can help your child paint a more balanced picture. Here are some things to say:

- "Great effort and improvement. Keep working hard, and winning will take care of itself."
- "That was a tough one to lose, but your defense showed improvement. Stay with it, and it'll pay off."
- "Really good effort. That's all anyone can ask. I'm proud of you."
- "It never feels good to lose, but you showed terrific sportsmanship. Way to go!"
- Ask your child, "Did you learn anything from this that you can apply in school and in other parts of your life?"

Above all, don't blame or get angry with the child. He or she feels bad enough already. Support and understanding, sincerely given, will be very helpful at this time. If, however, an athlete hasn't given maximum effort, communicate your unhappiness without putting down the youngster as a person. Athletes need to learn that effort is completely controllable and that they are accountable. Again, focus on the future and tell children that they owe it to themselves and their teammates to give maximum effort. Effort is a *decision*, not a trait.

Perhaps your young athlete plays on a team that loses regularly. If winning is the only goal that is set, your child will be constantly frustrated. If, on the other hand, scaled-down goals are developed, a sense of accomplishment can result as improvement occurs. Knowledgeable coaches often use individual and team goal-setting to create a kind of "game within the game." For example, the team objective may be to reduce the number of errors, strikeouts, fumbles, or penalties in the next few competitive events. Even if competitions are lost, children can experience a sense of accomplishment as they attain modified goals.

You can promote similar goal-setting on an individual level with your child. In addition to performance goals, you can place emphasis on such important ingredients to success as effort and teamwork. Many a team and many an athlete have been helped to feel as if progress was made toward a larger objective when they succeeded at smaller subgoals.

### How to Deal with a Winning Streak

Strangely enough, winning can create its own problems. One is overconfidence and being too cocky. Unless carefully handled, winning teams can become arrogant and disrespectful to teams they defeat.

When a win occurs the most natural thing is to enjoy it. Youngsters should be allowed to feel good about winning—they've earned it. But they should also be reminded to show consideration for their opponents. Emphasize that it never feels good to lose and there is no justification for rubbing it in. Instead, tell youngsters to be gracious winners and to give their opponents a pat on the back or a high five in a sincere manner.

---

The healthiest competition occurs when average people win by putting in above-average effort.

—*Colin Powell, former Secretary of State*

---

During a winning streak, most athletes experience not only the pleasure of winning but also the increased pressure not to lose. An additional danger is that if a team wins too regularly and too easily, they may get bored and take their success for granted. In such instances, a focus on effort and continued improvement can provide an additional and meaningful goal for youngsters. Here are some things to say if your child played well during the win:

- "Way to go! You showed a lot of effort and improvement. Keep it up."
- "You must feel satisfied with your effort and performance. I'm proud of you."
- "You met the challenge really well. Is there anything in your game that needs more work and improvement?"

If your child played badly, here are some things to say:

- "That was a good one to win. Is there any part of your game that needs work?"
- "Let's enjoy that win. Keep focusing on your effort and learning, and you'll do better next time."
- Ask your child, "Did you learn anything from this that you can apply in school and in other parts of your life?"

## PARENTAL BEHAVIOR AT PRACTICES AND COMPETITIONS

Much of the joy of being a youth sport parent comes from watching your child during practices and competitions. Most children also appreciate their parents' interest and attendance. What youngster isn't bolstered by looking up into the stands and seeing Mom and Dad in rapt attention?

Through their cooperative efforts, many parents are productive contributors to youngsters' sport experiences. But the negative effects of a rather small minority of parents are all too obvious. The following are extreme examples of media reports concerning parents engaging in criminally violent actions:

- In Massachusetts, a referee died after he was beaten unconscious following a hockey practice by a father who was upset about rough play in a scrimmage. The assailant was convicted of involuntary man-slaughter.

- At a Philadelphia-area youth football game, a player's father bran-dished a .357 magnum during a dispute with a coach over his son's playing time.
- A Long Island, New York, soccer mom angered over being dropped from the team e-mail list for game-day directions was arrested after slamming a metal folding chair across the face of her daughter's coach. The woman was charged with second-degree reckless endangerment.

Fortunately, such incidents are not the norm. The vast majority of parents do behave appropriately at youth sport events. But the minority who misbehave can spoil it for all the rest. It takes only a few incon-siderate parents to turn what should be a pleasant atmosphere into a nightmare for all concerned.

Although they may appear totally engrossed in the competition, many children are very sensitive to what is being said from the stands. Laughing or poking fun at an athlete who makes a mistake may inject some humor for the spectators, but it may be heartbreaking for the child. Likewise, "bench jockeying," or attempts to rattle the opposi-tion, is inappropriate at the youth sport level. Indeed, one can question whether such actions are in good taste at any level.

It is easy to get caught up in the action of the competition and to sud-denly find yourself verbally participating. Parents should never shout criticism or instruction at their children. This applies also to teammates and opponents. If you wish to shout encouragement or praise, make sure that your mastery approach extends to the other players as well. Again, codes of sportsmanship dictate that recognition also be given to opponents. There is no reason why a great play or a great effort made by the opposition should not also be appreciated.

Children are not the only ones who are the targets of barbed com-ments. Some onlookers seem to forget that youth sport programs could not exist without coaches and officials who give unselfishly of their time

## A LITTLE BOY

He stands at the plate with his heart pounding fast; the
    bases are loaded; the die has been cast.
Mom and Dad cannot help him; he stands all alone.
A hit at this moment would send the winning run home.
The ball nears the plate; he swings but he misses; there's a
    groan from the crowd with boos and some hisses.
A thoughtless voice shouts, "Strike out, you bum."
Tears fill his eyes; the game's no longer fun.
Remember, he's just a little boy who stands all alone.
So open your heart and give him a break; for it's moments
    like this a man you can make.
Keep this in mind when you hear someone shout.
Remember, he's still a little boy and not a man yet.

—Anonymous

and energy. They deserve your respect and support, and they should be
treated with dignity. As tempting as it may be, it is simply not appropriate to second-guess, yell instructions, or disagree with decisions made
by the coach.

It is as American as apple pie to boo and criticize judgments made
by sport officials. But such behavior has no place in youth sports! Officials are human, and they make mistakes. Like your child, they are
amateurs. The officials are honestly trying to do their best. Booing their
decisions will not change the outcome or improve the situation in any
way. Moreover, parents who "get on" officials provide very poor models
for their children, and such behavior can prove highly embarrassing to
the young athlete. Heckling poisons the atmosphere and drives officials
out of sports.

> Coaches, program directors, sport officials, and the
> athletes themselves have a right to demand that
> spectators conform to acceptable standards of behavior.

In addition to acknowledging some obviously inappropriate actions (using profanity, drinking alcohol, throwing objects, etc.), the following rules for parental behavior have been recommended by youth sport authorities:

- *Do* remain seated in the spectator area during the contest.
- *Don't* interfere with your child's coach. Parents must be willing to relinquish the responsibility for their child to the coach for the duration of the practice or competition.
- *Do* express interest, encouragement, and support to your child.
- *Don't* shout instructions or criticisms to the children.
- *Do* lend a hand when a coach or official asks for help.
- *Don't* make abusive comments to athletes, parents, officials, or coaches of either team.

These rules make good sense. There is also a *video rule* that is easy to remember. When you attend practices and competitions, imagine you are being videotaped. The two-part rule is simple:

- *Don't* do anything that would embarrass yourself or your child.
- *Do* things that would make your son or daughter proud.

What if a parent violates a rule of conduct? Good sportsmanship among spectators is a goal worth working for. Parents have the obligation not only to control their own behavior, but also to remind others of their responsibilities, if necessary. When parents behave badly (loud, rowdy, obnoxious actions), it is the duty of program administrators and sport officials to step in. But you can also help to correct the situation with a reminder that *"It's just kids playing a sport."*

A word of caution is warranted here: when parents misbehave, it could be emotionally charged and potentially dangerous. So be very careful and diplomatic in how you approach unruly parents.

## GETTING ALONG WITH YOUR CHILD'S COACH

Some of the most difficult problems that arise in youth sports involve the relationship between parents and coaches. Anytime another significant adult enters your child's world, it may require an adjustment on your part. First of all, as we mentioned in Chapter 1 ("Parents' Roles and Responsibilities"), you must be willing to put up with another potential hero. You must also be willing to give up some control and influence in an important area of your youngster's life. Taking a backseat to another adult even temporarily isn't always easy. But things can get even more complicated and challenging if you find yourself at odds with coaching decisions that affect your young athlete.

> Your responsibility for what happens to your child does not stop when he or she enters a sport program or joins a team.

As a parent you have every right to be involved in and to look out for your child's welfare. The tricky part comes in deciding how and to what extent it is appropriate for you to be involved. When does appropriate concern become interfering and meddling? At what point must your concern with the happiness and well-being of your child be tempered by respect and understanding for the role of the coach? What should you do if issues like the following spring up?

- Your child isn't getting to play enough during competitions.
- Your child is not playing the position best suited to his or her talents.
- The coach is mistreating youngsters either verbally or physically.
- The coach is engaging in inappropriate behavior, such as cursing or hazing of officials or opponents.
- The coach is using technically incorrect, questionable, or possibly dangerous coaching methods.

- The coach is demanding too much time or commitment from the youngsters, such that the sport is interfering with other activities.
- The coach is losing perspective of the purpose of youth sports and seems preoccupied with winning, thus putting additional stress on athletes.

Because each situation is somewhat unique, there are no cut-and-dried answers that apply to every case. Nonetheless, there are some general principles that can be helpful.

When incidents such as those listed above occur, it would be a mistake not to consider them worthy of attention. The best starting point is to view them as problems that you and the coach must work on together to resolve. The key to doing so is establishing communication and then keeping the lines of dialogue open.

Many parents first become aware of problems when their children complain about the coach. If this happens, several steps can be taken:

- Sit down with your youngster and get his or her point of view. Listen and express concern, but do not form a judgment or make condemning statements about the coach.
- After listening, you may decide that the issue does not require your involvement and that it might best be worked out by your youngster and the coach. You can help your child by giving suggestions on how to approach the coach and express concerns. If you can help resolve the issue without your direct involvement, your child may learn some very important interpersonal skills and gain confidence in his or her problem-solving ability.
- If the situation warrants it, contact the coach and indicate that you would like to have a conference. Such discussions should never occur during practices or competitions and should not include the child. Having your child there may put the coach on the defensive and create an adversary relationship between you and the coach. What is needed is a mutual problem-solving approach.

Communication is the key to friendly,
productive relations with coaches.

When you meet with the coach, try to create an open and receptive atmosphere for discussion:

- You can help create a positive environment by telling the coach that you appreciate his or her interest in the children and contributions to the program. You might also communicate that you understand how demanding the role of a coach is.
- Next, indicate that there is an issue that you would like to discuss and that if there is a problem, you would like to work with the coach in resolving it. Here are some examples of ways in which you can introduce the problem:

   Sean told me that he would like to get to play more during games. He feels that since he comes to every practice and tries hard, he'd like to get to play more. (Note that the coach is not being directly accused of not playing Sean enough, which might create defensiveness. Whenever possible, frame the problem in terms of a positive goal to be achieved.)

   I have been to several of your basketball practices, and I have seen the drill where you have the kids practice taking charging fouls and being run over by an offensive player. I am concerned about the possibility of injury. Is there a safer drill that could be substituted?

   I've seen some of the kids get very upset after being yelled at, and I am concerned. I wonder if there isn't some way of making it more fun for the kids. Sometimes we adults don't realize how easy it can be to hurt feelings.

   Kristin joined the program because she wanted to have fun and because she enjoys playing softball. There seems to be such an emphasis on winning and so much pressure put on the girls to perform that at least for Kristin, it's becoming stressful rather than constructive.

- After expressing your concern, you might once again acknowledge what a difficult job coaching is, but say that you thought the coach would want to hear about your concern because you believe he or she has the best interests of the children at heart.

- Then tell the coach that you would like to hear his or her view of the situation. Again, the emphasis should be on resolving the problem together.

---

**Communication is a two-way street.
It involves listening as well as expressing.**

---

You will need to be prepared to listen honestly and openly to the coach's point of view. For example, his or her opinion of your child's ability and deserved playing time may be somewhat different from your own. And the role of coach requires that he or she make a judgment about playing time.

Parents who voice their concerns are often surprised when they are asked to participate in a solution to the problem. For example, a father who disagreed with the coach's way of teaching a particular skill was asked by the coach to assume the position of assistant coach. The coach acknowledged that he had little experience in that particular area and that he would appreciate the father's assistance. In another instance, a mother who expressed concern that her son was not playing enough was asked by the coach to play catch with the son so that he would improve enough to play more. Thus, you must sometimes be prepared to contribute time and effort—as well as your opinion.

In some cases, you may find that it isn't possible to correct the situation with the coach. If you feel strongly enough about the issue and are convinced that the coach's actions affect the physical or psychological well-being of the children, you may need to take further action. Several options are available:

- First, you may appeal to a higher authority. If a coach is being abusive to children, for example, this should be brought to the attention of league administrators.

- If the issue concerns only your child and not others, the solution may be to request a transfer to another team and coach.
- The last, most drastic, and least desirable alternative may be to remove your child from the program. This should always be a last resort because it may have some negative consequences of its own. For example, the child may be called a quitter.

Fortunately, most coaches are firmly committed to providing the best possible experiences for youngsters. When approached properly, they will usually be open to parents' concerns and motivated to deal effectively with problems.

> Coaches deserve respect, encouragement, support, and appreciation from parents.

Up to now, we have been focusing on undesirable things that might come to your attention. But relating to your child's coach goes beyond this. When things are going well, be sure to provide reinforcement to the coach. This adult is playing an important role in your child's life. All too often, the only feedback coaches get from parents is negative. It is important to let them know when they are doing a good job. They truly deserve it!

### GIVING ATTENTION TO THE NONATHLETE IN THE FAMILY

Children who are heavily involved or gifted in athletics have no problem in getting lots of attention. In some families, so much attention is paid to the star athlete that brothers and sisters may fade into the background. This is most likely to happen when parents are heavily invested in sports themselves and prize athletic accomplishments. It is important to keep in mind that *all children need attention, love, and support from parents.* When nonathletes feel ignored, parents may find themselves having to deal with jealousy, feelings of rejection, and lowered self-esteem.

> Find something special in each
> of your children to love and celebrate.

Although involvement in sports is to be encouraged and valued, other areas of achievement should be given equal billing. The nonathletic brother who is trying hard in school or who is musically inclined or who has a knack for making friends deserves recognition and support just as the athlete does. Clearly communicate that each child has unique gifts and endearing qualities and that you are aware of them. Also emphasize that growing up involves finding out which things youngsters are best at and enjoy most. Approval of each child as an individual lays the foundation for self-acceptance in all of your children.

> All children deserve quality time with their parents.

Your involvement with your athletic son or daughter may vary in degree, but it will almost certainly require a time commitment on your part. This should not detract from personal time with the nonathletic children in your family. How can you ensure that all of your children are getting attention?

- Keep a daily record of the amount of time spent with each child over a two-week period. You might be surprised to find a huge amount of time is spent on the activities of the young athlete.
- Block special time around activities and interests of your other children. When this is done, no child in the family will feel left out.

**PROTECTING YOUR CHILD: BULLYING AND SEXUAL ABUSE**
If there's anything that gives parents sleepless nights, it's the thought that their child might experience some form of abuse. Whether the

child is the victim, witness, or perpetrator, it's hard to get the thought of bullying and sexual abuse out of your mind. What can you do if you suspect your child is being abused? And better yet, what can be done to prevent it? We address these questions in this section.

### Bullying

Bullying is repeated aggressive behavior that can be physical, verbal (name-calling, taunting, insulting), or relational. Bullying is a serious problem that has harmful effects on both the victim and the bully. Boys frequently bully using physical threats and actions, while girls are more likely to engage in relationship bullying, which includes refusing to talk to someone, excluding the victim from a group or activity, or spreading lies or rumors about the child. Bullying can occur in virtually any setting, including the sport environment. Social media have magnified the problem, with the Internet enabling an epidemic of cyberbullying that can follow a child into his or her home, which would otherwise be a safe haven.

Regardless of the form it takes, bullying takes a terrible emotional and physical toll on many children. Victims of bullying feel hurt, angry, afraid, helpless, hopeless, isolated, and ashamed. They may even feel guilty that the bullying is somehow their fault. Victims of bullying are at greater risk of developing mental health problems such as depression, anxiety, and low self-esteem. When it occurs in sport settings, victims are more likely to miss, skip, or drop out of sports to avoid being bullied. Moreover, the scars inflicted by bullying can persist long into the future and can predispose a young person to develop psychological problems in adulthood.

---

Bullying is not a form of conflict; it is a form of victimization.

—*Dr. Gabriela Reed, pediatric psychologist, Children's Medical Center of Dallas*

---

Because of its pervasiveness and harmful consequences, parents should discuss bullying with their children. They should open the lines of communication to find out if anyone is treating their child or any other child badly and, if necessary, should take steps to stop the abuse. Simply talking about the problem can be a huge stress reliever for a child who's being bullied:

- Be supportive and listen to a child's feelings without judgment, criticism, or blame.
- Don't minimize the child's feelings or tell the child that he or she should simply ignore or shrug off the bullying unless the child is capable of doing so (and few children are).
- Try to find out if your child is doing anything to evoke negative responses and dislike from others. Aside from children who come across as anxious, socially awkward, insincere, and withdrawn, those who are annoying, argumentative, and aggressive are also targets of bullying. If your child fits into these victim categories, counsel your child on how to change the offending behavior and become more socially successful.

Children who engage or participate in bullying also deserve attention. If you find that your child is a party to bullying, make sure he or she understands how hurtful such behavior can be. Foster empathy by encouraging your child to look at his or her actions from the victim's perspective, and how it would feel to be treated in that manner.

In sports, adult supervisors should make sure that bullying does not occur. An emphasis on team-building and creating a "family" atmosphere on a sport team can reduce the chances that bullying will occur and create a cohesive team experience that will benefit everyone. If you witness bullying or hazing in the sport setting (whether the target is your child or not), arrange a conference with the coach to communicate what you've seen or heard about and ask the coach to take measures to stop the abuse. If the coach is unresponsive to your request, communicate your concerns to the program administrator. Any quality sport program will want to promote a positive, fun, and growth-inducing setting for young athletes, and bullying has no place in such a program.

## Sexual Abuse

If the psychological scars from bullying are painful, the long-term emotional and psychological damage resulting from sexual abuse can be devastating and almost always requires psychological treatment to undo the damage. Child sexual abuse involves any sexual activity with a child where consent is not or cannot be given. This includes sexual contact that is accomplished by force or threat of force, regardless of the age of the participants, and all sexual contact between an adult and a child, regardless of whether or not the child understands the sexual nature of the activity. The sexually abusive acts may include sexual penetration, sexual touching, or noncontact sexual acts such as exposure or voyeurism (for example, ogling of the child's body or exposing a child to pornography).

> Children of all races, ethnicities, cultures, and economic backgrounds are vulnerable to sexual abuse.

Even psychologists and psychiatrists used to think that sexual abuse of children was quite rare. We now know differently. Sexual abuse occurs far more commonly than most people realize. Research summarized by the U.S. Centers for Disease Control and Prevention indicates that approximately one in six boys and one in four girls are sexually abused before the age of 18. Most victims suffer the abuse at the hands of someone they know, often a trusted adult. It can occur inside or outside the home. Ironically, the same factors that create a nurturing environment and foster positive personal growth can also open the doors to sexually abusive behaviors. Pedophiles are often drawn to positive youth settings, such as teaching, scouting, or sports, because such settings bring them into contact with so many potential targets. Youth sport organizations are increasingly aware that they must balance their goal of nurturing and caring for children with the need to keep youth safe.

As well-publicized events involving coaches suggest, parents and sport administrators must be vigilant because the tiny minority of abusers who find their way into youth sport positions can do untold damage. Contact between coaches and children should be regulated so as to minimize the chances that any child can be victimized. For example, many organizations prohibit coaches from being alone with children, being in the shower room with them after events, or driving children home without the parents' permission. They should require more than one coach to be present on road trips or other events away from home. Many coaches who felt perfectly natural patting children on the behind or hugging them are now limiting themselves to high fives, fist bumps, and verbal praise so as to avoid any signs of impropriety.

Experts on child abuse recommend that parents reduce the likelihood of abuse by educating their children about what is and is not permissible adult behavior. Even young children can understand the "swimsuit" guideline that it is never OK for an adult to touch the child in the areas covered by a swimsuit. Parents should tell their child: "If someone tries to touch your body and do things that make you feel funny, say NO to that person and tell me right away." They should also tell their child that respect for authority does not mean doing everything a teacher, babysitter, or coach tells you to do if it seems wrong. Above all, keep the lines of communication open with your child so that if the worst should ever happen, the child will tell you about it. In a variety of ways, child sexual abusers can make victims fearful of telling anyone about what's happening, and only when a special effort is made to help the child to feel safe can he or she talk freely. It is a tragedy that many victims undergo long-term abuse and suffer in silence because they cannot confide in those who would protect them.

Parents should be attentive to sudden changes in their child's behavior that may reflect a traumatic event. This may include an increase in nightmares or other sleeping difficulties, angry outbursts or aggressive behavior, anxiety, depression, withdrawn behavior, difficulty walking or sitting, or a desire to avoid certain people or situations (which could include wanting to quit sports). Children who have undergone abuse often feel damaged or worthless, so be attentive to an apparent decrease in self-esteem.

What should you do if your child tells you he or she has been sexually abused? Obviously, this would be very disturbing to any parent and how you react is critical to the child's ability to resolve and heal the trauma of sexual abuse. The American Psychological Association provides important information on child abuse and suggests the following guidelines:

- Encourage the child to talk freely, and don't make judgmental comments. Find out specifically what happened and when.
- Show that you understand and take seriously what the child is saying. Children who are listened to and understood have a much better outcome than those who are not.
- Assure the child that they did the right thing in telling. A child who is close to the abuser may feel guilty about revealing the secret or frightened if the abuser has threatened to harm the child or other family members as punishment for telling the secret.
- Tell the child that he or she is not to blame for the sexual abuse. In attempting to make sense out of the abuse, many victims believe that somehow they caused it. Some may even view it as a form of punishment for imagined or real wrongdoings.
- Finally, offer the child emotional support and protection, and promise that you will promptly take steps to see that the abuse stops.

If you suspect that abuse has occurred, it is not your job to investigate or to take vengeance on the perpetrator. Instead, you should report it immediately to the local police or district attorney's office. Reports (and the identity of those making them) are confidential and people who report possible or actual abuse in good faith are immune from prosecution. The agency will investigate the abuse and take action to protect your child and, given evidence of abuse, prosecute the offender.

Finally, parents should consult with their family doctor or pediatrician. Your doctor may refer the child to a medical specialist in evaluating and treating sexual abuse. The specialist will conduct a physical examination and treat any physical damage from the abuse, gather evidence concerning the abuse, and provide reassurance to the child.

## HELPING YOUR MARRIAGE SURVIVE YOUTH SPORTS

With respect to the quality of family life, youth sports can be an important element in promoting growth and solidarity. When parents share significant experiences with their children, stronger bonds can be forged not only between the parents and children but also between the parents themselves. The sport environment is a place where you and your spouse can actually witness and enjoy the growth and development of your child. You cannot sit in a classroom and watch academic skills blossom. But you can have a sideline seat to the development of your child's athletic and social skills. We strongly encourage you to take advantage of this significant window of opportunity.

As you are well aware, children place certain strains on marriage. Children are very needy, and your attention and devotion are the foundation of good parenting. Each phase through which a child develops places different pressures and requirements on you and your spouse. As a result, parents find that they have less time for themselves and for their spouses. Just as youth sports can be a double-edged sword to the athlete, they can also affect husband-wife relationships in a positive or a negative way. Couples need to be aware of this fact and to be prepared to counteract the potential pitfalls.

> Children not only are a blessing but also
> offer special challenges to a marriage.

Many couples center their lives on children and are unaware that their relationship is remaining static or perhaps even crumbling from lack of attention. Such couples unwittingly drift apart during the child-rearing years only to find at the midlife crisis that they have little left in common except their children. The husbands and wives now find that they have become "married singles." They become absorbed in their day-to-day activities and come to discover that the excitement of their earlier years together has died. On the surface, all appears tranquil. The serenity comes from a lack of awareness of what is missing in the relationship. The escalating divorce rate and the number of single-parent families provide grim evidence of this.

For some couples, youth sports become a deceptive blessing. Such couples avoid facing problems in their marriage through their children's sport involvement. The focus of their lives becomes the child in the athletic arena, and they become so wrapped up in his or her activities that they avoid dealing with marital discord.

Along with increased financial obligations, your child's entry into a youth sport program will likely place greater demands on your marriage. As parents discover, time commitments expand due to such things as driving children to and from practices and competitions, participating on parent committees, or serving as coaches. Some parents find to their dismay that practices are held during the dinner hour and that their kitchen becomes a cafeteria with several shifts. The fun and togetherness of family meals become a thing of the past. For most families, this is only a seasonal happening. But for families whose youngsters are heavily involved in sports, this becomes the normal pattern of living.

> Marital bliss doesn't just happen automatically;
> it comes from actively working at it.

Perhaps the most important thing is to decide exactly what your priorities are and what you want out of the sport experience, not only for your child but also for the rest of the family. If your priorities are to grow closer as a family, then you need to think of ways in which you can use sports to improve and not damage this process. In most instances, you will have to balance the negative against the positive things that your child and the family might experience in a sport program. Be aware of what is likely to be required and how much time and effort you are willing to devote. Once into a program, you should also keep in mind that you can easily be seduced into more and more involvement. For example, you will have to take your turn in carpooling, and you may be asked to perform other duties. Before you know it, your responsibilities can snowball.

What do couples do, then, to compensate for the demands that youth sports can make on their relationship? Here are some tips for dealing with the special challenges of being youth sport husbands and wives:

- As mentioned earlier, find ways to spend adequate time with all your children, particularly those who are not involved in sports.
- Likewise, it is important for spouses to devote time to their own relationship. Private moments spent away from the children can serve to maintain and invigorate your marriage. Recreational pursuits for you and your spouse, an occasional weekend away by yourselves, dinners out, and a cultivation of interests you share in common can help maintain the sparkle in your marriage.
- All couples must continue to find ways to improve communication. Get into the habit of talking regularly about your thoughts and, especially, your feelings. As long as the lines of communication are kept open and problems openly discussed, your relationship with your loved ones can not only endure, but deepen.

# Bibliography

American Psychological Association. (2012). *Child sexual abuse: What parents should know*. Retrieved from http://wwwa.pa.org/pi/families/resources/child-sexual-abuse.aspx.

Brustad, R. J., & Parker, M. (2005). Enhancing positive youth development through sport and physical activity. *Psychologica, 39,* 75–93.

Clark, N. (2008). *Nancy Clark's sports nutrition guidebook* (4th ed.). Champaign, IL: Human Kinetics.

Cumming, S. P., Smoll, F. L., Smith, R. E., & Grossbard, J. R. (2007). Is winning everything? The relative contributions of motivational climate and won-lost percentage in youth sports. *Journal of Applied Sport Psychology, 19,* 322–336.

Greendorfer, S. L., Lewko, J. H., & Rosengren, K. S. (2002). Family and gender-based influences in sport socialization of children and adolescents. In F. L. Smoll & R. E. Smith (Eds.), *Children and youth in sport: A biopsychosocial perspective* (2nd ed., pp. 153–186). Dubuque, IA: Kendall/Hunt.

Horn, T. S., & Horn, J. L. (2007). Family influences on children's sport and physical activity participation, behavior, and psychosocial responses. In G. Tenenbaum & R. C. Eklund (Eds.), *Handbook of sport psychology* (3rd ed., pp. 685–711). Hoboken, NJ: Wiley.

Malina, R. M., Bouchard, C., & Bar-Or, O. (2004). *Growth, maturation, and physical activity* (2nd ed.). Champaign, IL: Human Kinetics.

Malina, R. M., & Clark, M. A. (Eds.). (2003). *Youth sports: Perspectives for a new century*. Monterey, CA: Coaches Choice.

Micheli, L. J., & Jenkins, M. (2001). *The sports medicine bible for young athletes*. Naperville, IL: Sourcebooks.

National Collegiate Athletic Association. (2011a). *Estimated probability of competing in athletics beyond the high school interscholastic level*. Retrieved from http://ncaa.org/wps/wcm/connect/public/NCAA/Issues/Recruiting/Probability+of+Going+Pro.

National Collegiate Athletic Association. (2011b). *Guide for the college-bound student-athlete*. Retrieved from http://www.ncaapublications.com/productdownloads/CBSA.pdf.

National Council of Youth Sports. (2008). *Report on trends and participation in organized youth sports*. Retrieved from http://www.ncys.org/publications/2008-sports-participation-study.php.

National Federation of State High School Associations. (2011). *2010–2011 High school athletics participation survey*. Retrieved from http://www.nfhs.org/contact.aspx?id=3282.

Roberts, G. C., Treasure, D. C., & Conroy, D. E. (2007). Understanding the dynamics of motivation in sport and physical activity: An achievement goal interpretation. In G. Tenenbaum & R. C. Eklund (Eds.), *Handbook of sport psychology* (3rd ed., pp. 3–30). New York: Wiley.

Scanlan, T. K., Babkes, M. L., & Scanlan, L. A. (2005). Participation in sport: A developmental glimpse at emotion. In J. L. Mahoney, R. W. Larson, & J. S. Eccles (Eds.), *Organized activities as contexts of development: Extracurricular activities, after-school and community programs* (pp. 275–309). Mahwah, NJ: Erlbaum.

Smith, N. J., & Worthington-Roberts, B. (1989). *Food for sport*. Palo Alto, CA: Bull.

Smith, R. E., & Smoll, F. L. (2011). Cognitive-behavioral coach training: A translational approach to theory, research, and intervention. In J. K. Luiselli & D. D. Reed (Eds.), *Behavioral sport psychology: Evidence-based approaches to performance enhancement* (pp. 227–248). New York, NY: Springer.

Smith, R. E., & Smoll, F. L. (2012). *Sport psychology for youth coaches: Developing champions in sports and life.* Lanham, MD: Rowman & Littlefield.

Smith, R. E., Smoll, F. L., & O'Rourke, D. J. (2011). Anxiety management. In T. Morris & P. Terry (Eds.), *The new sport and exercise psychology companion* (pp. 227–255). Morgantown, WV: Fitness Information Technology.

Smoll, F. L., Cumming, S. P., & Smith, R. E. (2011). Enhancing coach-parent relationships in youth sports: Increasing harmony and minimizing hassle. *International Journal of Sports Science & Coaching, 6,* 13–26.

Smoll, F. L., & Smith, R. E. (Eds.). (2002). *Children and youth in sport: A biopsychosocial perspective* (2nd ed.). Dubuque, IA: Kendall/Hunt.

Smoll, F. L., & Smith, R. E. (Producers). (2009a). *Mastery approach to coaching: A self-instruction program for youth sport coaches* [DVD]. Seattle, WA: Youth Enrichment in Sports.

Smoll, F. L., & Smith, R. E. (Producers). (2009b). *Mastery approach to parenting in sports: A self-instruction program for youth sport parents* [DVD]. Seattle, WA: Youth Enrichment in Sports.

Smoll, F. L., & Smith, R. E. (2010). Conducting psychologically oriented coach-training programs: A social-cognitive approach. In J. M. Williams (Ed.), *Applied sport psychology: Personal growth to peak performance* (6th ed., pp. 392–416). Boston: McGraw-Hill.

White, S. A. (2007). Parent-created motivational climate. In S. Jowett & D. Lavallee (Eds.), *Social psychology in sport* (pp. 131–143). Champaign, IL: Human Kinetics.

# Index

# About the Authors

**Frank L. Smoll** is professor of psychology and a member of the Center for Child and Family Well-Being at the University of Washington. Dr. Smoll's research focuses on coaching behaviors in youth sports and on the psychological effects of competition on children and adolescents. He has published more than 130 scientific articles and book chapters, and he has coauthored/edited 22 books and manuals on children's athletics. Professor Smoll is a fellow of the American Psychological Association, the National Academy of Kinesiology, and the Association for Applied Sport Psychology (AASP). Dr. Smoll is an AASP Certified Consultant and was the recipient of AASP's Distinguished Professional Practice Award. As an undergraduate, he played on championship basketball and baseball teams, and he is a member of the Ripon College Athletic Hall of Fame. In the area of applied sport psychology, Dr. Smoll has extensive experience in conducting psychologically oriented coaching clinics and workshops for parents of young athletes.

**Ronald E. Smith** is professor of psychology and director of the Clinical Psychology Training Program at the University of Washington. He has also served as head of the social psychology and personality area and as codirector of the sport psychology graduate program. Professor Smith's major research interests are in personality, stress and coping, and performance enhancement research and intervention. He has published more than 200 scientific articles and book chapters, and he has authored or coauthored 34 books. Dr. Smith is a fellow of the American Psychological Association, a past president of the Association for Applied Sport Psychology, and the recipient of a Distinguished Alumnus Award from the UCLA Neuropsychiatric Institute for his contributions to the field of mental health. For twelve years, he directed a psychological skills training program for the Houston Astros and has served as team counselor for the Seattle Mariners and as a training consultant to the Oakland Athletics and to Major League Soccer.